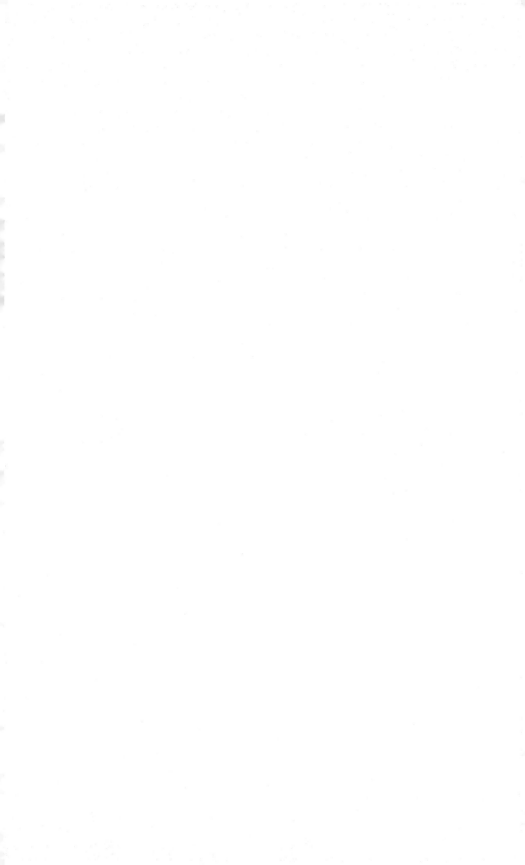

A TIME FOR
Miracles

Finding Your Way through the Wilderness of Alzheimer's

KATHLEEN BROWN

WestBow
PRESS®
A DIVISION OF THOMAS NELSON
& ZONDERVAN

WestBow Press books may be ordered through booksellers or by contacting:

WestBow Press
A Division of Thomas Nelson & Zondervan
1663 Liberty Drive
Bloomington, IN 47403
www.westbowpress.com
844-714-3454

All Scripture quotations are taken from the Holy Bible, NEW
INTERNATIONAL VERSION®, NIV® Copyright © 1973, 1978, 1984, 2011
by Biblica, Inc.® Used by permission. All rights reserved worldwide.

ISBN: 979-8-3850-4207-4 (sc)
ISBN: 979-8-3850-4206-7 (e)

Library of Congress Control Number: 2025900665

Print information available on the last page.

WestBow Press rev. date: 1/29/2025

With thanks and love to my husband, Harold.
Though his name is seldom mentioned,
he was always there
with his strength,
his wisdom,
his love.
Always.

The desert and the parched land will be glad;
The wilderness will rejoice and blossom…
Strengthen the feeble hands, Steady the knees that give way;
Say to those with fearful hearts,
"Be strong, do not fear; Your God will come…
He will come to save you."
Then will the eyes of the blind be opened
And the ears of the deaf unstopped.
Then will the lame leap like a deer,
And the mute tongue shout for joy.
Water will gush forth in the wilderness
And streams in the desert…
And a highway will be there;
It will be called the Way of Holiness…
And those the Lord has rescued will return…
Gladness and joy will overtake them,
And sorrow and sighing will flee away.
—Is. 35:1, 3–6, 8, 10, NIV

Contents

Foreword

This is a book of hope.

Caring for a loved one with dementia requires time, energy, love, patience, and a great deal of sacrifice. However, there are miracles and laughter on this journey as well. There is much to be thankful for, as you will find in this book.

Alzheimer's disease (AD) is characterized by amnesia, loss of language skills, loss of functional motor skills, cognitive and recognition capability and executive function. Not only does one lose the ability to recognize family and friends, but also the power to judge the importance of certain tasks, like paying bills; the capability to perform basic calculations; and the ability to plan or sequence tasks. One can get lost while driving in familiar neighborhoods. Street lights and signs lose their meaning. Operating appliances, balancing a checkbook and cooking a meal become challenging obstacles and even familiar recipes are forgotten.

In later stages, bathing, table manners and personal hygiene are forgotten. Keeping patients clean, dry and fed becomes an increasingly difficult burden for caregivers. As the disease progresses, Alzheimer's patients may try to wear the same clothes day after day. Clothes inappropriate for the weather are sometimes chosen, for example, winter clothes in summer. Personal grooming is less important to the patient and becomes a source of conflict. Attempts to assist the patient in bathing or grooming can provoke anxiety or anger.

This book explores the role of family and caregivers and their struggles to cope with the highs and lows of a loved one with AD. There is hardship, but many periods of happiness and satisfaction along the way.

The prevalence of mild to moderate AD in the United States is estimated at 6.9 million. By 2050, it is estimated that a new case of AD will be diagnosed every thirty-three seconds. The symptoms typically begin several years before the diagnosis is made. It progresses as a slow gradual decline in cognition. Family members may notice mild trouble with recall of words or previous conversations. Often this is written off to "normal aging." Eventually the deficits become more noticeable and worrisome. The spouse will often fill in the memory gaps for their impaired mate, functioning as an "auxiliary brain."

As the disease progresses, family roles change. Spouses learn to take on the tasks/roles of their partners with AD. When adult children are available, these tasks may be shared to lessen the burden on the healthy parent. Role reversal also occurs when children assume care of their affected parent. This transition can be smooth or rocky depending upon the individuals involved as well as the ability and patience of the caregiver.

As a geriatric psychiatrist, I treat patients with Alzheimer's disease to try to improve their cognition, behavior and functional skills. Behavior issues range from depression and anxiety to paranoia and aggression. Hallucinations and delusions are sometimes present as well.

Irritability, restlessness and agitation make caring for these patients more complicated. Medication is only a small part of the treatment plan. Educating caregivers in how to manage this behavior is more impactful. The tips found in this book can help ease this burden as caregivers provide the bulk of the treatment. These "front-line soldiers" are responsible for maintaining a safe, comfortable environment for their loved ones with AD. In addition to treating patients with AD, I also treat caregivers for depression, anxiety and "burnout." So many of them sacrifice so much for their parents or spouses that they put their own health at risk.

This book describes the sacrifices Kathleen Brown and her father made to care for her mother. It also shows how patience, faith and love can make this possible.

The choice of placement is a difficult one for families and it generally happens late in the illness when all in-home care options are exhausted. Physical limitations of caregivers, failing health of the patient or caregivers and complicated treatment regimens are among the reasons for placement. Behavior can also be a reason. Agitation, aggression or a marked irritability lead to caregiver burnout. Additionally, patient wandering and the inability for caregivers to maintain a safe environment may necessitate placement in a controlled setting. Typically, patients feel they are going to work or to a childhood home. Usually they don't recall their retirement or where home is.

My hope is that you will find this book as uplifting as I have. The stories and tips can help manage the burden of caring for these sometimes difficult loved ones. Love, patience, humor and compassion are key to dealing with this very human transition. However, the journey is not without fulfillment.

—Stephen F. Vobach, M.D.

Introduction

I discovered my mother's illness in the middle of a September trip from Texas to Colorado. I was traveling with my parents to visit my son who had recently graduated from college. As we drove west, Mom's bizarre behavior became more and more pronounced, until I could no longer rationalize or ignore it.

Although I didn't realize it until weeks later, I was joining my parents on a journey they had begun about five years earlier—the journey through the wilderness that is Alzheimer's disease.

In the beginning, I felt as if I'd been pulled into a black hole, with my mother far ahead of me, plunging into the bottomless void. I imagined my father falling beside her, near enough to touch her hand but not able to grasp it. I saw myself following them down, fast and straight, unable to help but unwilling to let them fall alone.

In real life, miracles broke our fall. Miracles put earth back under our feet and turned the whirling chaos of Alzheimer's into a path we could walk, often stumbling, but together. Around us, the land was a dark unknown, not unlike the great bottomless hole I had first imagined. But it was not a void. And it was not black. Miracles, big and small, lit our path through the wilderness of Alzheimer's.

At the time, my father was eighty-one. He looked and acted no older than seventy—healthy, squarely built, vigorous in thought and action. His one weakness was the macular degeneration that was stealing his eyesight. My mother was seventy-eight. She looked and acted at least ten years older, frail and unsteady, afraid and depressed. For over fifty years, their devotion to each other had enabled them to face life as a team of two-become-one; now Alzheimer's threatened to pull my mother down a path where my father couldn't follow.

I was forty-nine. My husband and I, married almost thirty years, had raised three sons who were grown and on their own. I had just been laid off from my job when I discovered my mother's illness. For six months, I took care of my parents by day and looked for employment at night. When the job offer finally came, I knew I'd been kidding myself to think my parents could manage without help. I declined the offer.

Mom was beyond realizing she was ill, but Dad and I desperately sought a diagnosis, some answers, hope. *Alzheimer's* was the last word we wanted to hear. We made an appointment with a psychiatrist; my mother refused to go. Wild-eyed, arms waving, she searched for something, anything, to convince us of her determination to go to "No doctor but mine!"—meaning my parents' primary care physician. Finding nothing handy to throw at us, she simply screamed.

So Dad and I went without her. Sitting in the cool calm of the doctor's office, we described my mother's symptoms as best we could, making certain the doctor understood that at times she acted just like her old self, her normal self. His response was similar to the one we received later from the primary care doctor. Their concurrence was as close as we ever came to getting an official diagnosis.

"Mr. Bailey," the psychiatrist said to my father, "I think you need to consider the possibility—the probability—that your wife has Alzheimer's."

He spoke gently, but his words hit with the impact of a fist to the stomach. Beyond those words, he gave us one more piece of advice—he suggested a book, *The 36-Hour Day.* We bought it that afternoon.

The 36-Hour Day was and still is widely accepted as one of the most helpful and informative books available about caring for someone with Alzheimer's. I found it difficult, however, to get past the title. The title told me, "Your future will be filled with impossible tasks, impossible challenges, impossibly long days." It said "hopeless."

So I put *The 36-Hour Day* aside for a while and we set out on our journey through Alzheimer's without a guidebook. There was nothing predictable about any stage of the trip. At no point during the last ten years of her life did we have any real certainty about my mother's physical or mental status. Because my father kept my mother's odd behavior to himself for as long as possible, he traveled alone for the first five of those years. We traveled together, he and I, for the last five.

Well, somewhat together. We traveled in the same direction and with the same intentions: to guide my mother, protect her, and do all in our power to help her enjoy life. But our paths were widely divergent when it came to methods. Dad's itinerary called for a private trip: no help from strangers, few stops to ask for directions. He just forged ahead into the darkness, determined to show that nothing had changed—he and Mom could manage as they always had. He accepted no help from anyone except me and my sister, who was rarely available. So what Dad saw as the all-important preservation of privacy became, for me, isolation.

The truth was that he and Mom could *not* manage as they always had. They needed help, more expert help than I could provide. How to convince him that he had options, how to make him see other ways of caring that would still preserve their life together at home—those were conversations I avoided, to my parents' detriment and my own.

Questions. The road was paved with them. What did we find as we searched for answers? Hard realities. Sad truths.

And miracles.

As we wound along the dark path through the deep forest of Alzheimer's, we found guideposts and warm cottages where we could rest. We found shortcuts and scenic byways. We traveled through times, places, and events of almost unbearable sadness, but we were also refreshed by moments of humor, when laughter rang loud and true.

And despite my father's determination that we needed no help, we met kind people along the way. Some were fellow travelers, some were professional guides, but most seemed to have been waiting along the path, just for us, ready to help, encourage, sympathize, or simply smile. They were the biggest miracles of all, the ones for whom we were most grateful.

That's what this book is about—miracles. It will tell with laughter and pain how miracles enabled us to cope with the everchanging challenges of Alzheimer's and how they helped us enjoy the last years of my mother's life.

I remember how desperate I was for practical information and tips, so I've included notes at the end of each chapter, along with a final section that describes more of the things we learned as we cared for Mom. I pray you can apply these suggestions directly to your own situation, or use them to prime the pump of your personal insight and experience.

And I hope you can laugh with us along the way. The humor that often surprised us as we rounded a corner will be on your path as well, another light for your way, like the sun peeking through on a cloudy day.

Most of all, I pray you find *hope* in these pages. I pray you see a hand extended to hold on to as you walk, so you can look up from the bumpy road and see the beauty along the way. Trust me—the road is difficult, but in that rough terrain, you will see where wisdom lives, and love.

Be watchful! This is a time for miracles.

Hitting the Road

Listen to me...you whom I have...carried since you were born. Even to your old age and gray hairs I am he, I am he who will sustain you. I have made you and I will carry you; I will sustain you and I will rescue you.
—ISAIAH 46:3–4, NIV

My mother's eyes were narrow and hot. Her cries ricocheted around the room, threatening to topple the thin beige walls of the little apartment. With one bare foot she kicked at my father's stomach as he faced her, holding her shoulders to keep her seated on the brown hand-me-down couch. Given the chance, she would have sprung at him like something wild, enraged.

"Marie! Marie!" my father shouted, his voice even louder than her growls.

I bent dangerously close to her flying hands, trying to make her see me, hear me. "Mama! That's Daddy! It's Daddy!" I fully expected the apartment manager or the police or both to show up any minute. Perhaps they were already there, knocking, banging, only we couldn't hear them.

It was September, a change of season, the beginning of fall. It was the month I discovered my mother had Alzheimer's.

I had lost my job earlier that month. A company reorganization meant my "services were no longer necessary." Not a catastrophe. As I thought about starting the search for new employment, I decided to take a break first, maybe a trip, only a week or so. My youngest son, Mark,

1

had just graduated from college in Colorado; I could take my parents to see his new place. His first solo apartment. They'd love that—a road trip in early autumn. Maybe the aspen would still be dancing like fire up the valleys and sliding golden down the mountains. It was as far as I could imagine from my old chaotic schedule of software sales. And this trip would give me the chance to spend some relaxing time with my parents.

I spent a lot of time with my mother while my three sons were growing up. Then Dad retired after thirty-four years as a tooling engineer with an aeronautical manufacturing company. At last, he and Mom were free to spend all their time together. They traveled occasionally, but mostly enjoyed their homes—the pink brick house where they raised my sister and me, and the more recently purchased home on a nearby lake. My parents were always content to be alone together, so much so that they had no close friends and little contact with relatives beyond my sister and me and our families.

When my sons were older, I went to work; time with my parents shrank even more. Although I lived only a short distance away from them, my life as a working mother didn't allow long, leisurely visits. I hoped this trip to Colorado would help us catch up with one another.

As I talked to Dad about the trip, his hesitation to jump at the opportunity should have sounded a warning, telling me, at the very least, that their love of travel had changed during the last couple of years. But I heard no bells. I only heard my father say, "I just can't plan things anymore. I never know when your mother's going to change her mind." He agreed to check with her—cautioned me not to expect anything, but he'd see.

His deference to her didn't surprise me. Putting her desires ahead of his had always been his style, his choice. Both of them were accustomed to things working that way. With 20/20 hindsight, I can see the changes that took place in Mom during the years just prior to that September, things I missed at the time or managed to ignore. Like her moodiness and unpredictability. Like my father answering the telephone and her not wanting to talk, a complete reversal of roles. She wanted to stay home more, eat out less, visit less, exercise less. Any differences I did notice in those years I had attributed to age. Mom was seventy-eight but acted ninety-eight. By contrast, Dad was eighty-one but looked and acted more like seventy. He had eyesight problems and she had high blood pressure, but both were relatively healthy.

So while I waited for their answer—well, Mom's answer— to my invitation, I told myself she had just grown old ahead of my father. Slower, more sedentary, more irritable. Maybe this trip would perk her up. I heard the longing in Dad's voice as he talked about the route, the weather, the scenery and, most of all, seeing Mark. Maybe Mom would hear it, too.

The next week found the three of us in their car heading west from Dallas toward Colorado. We drove a familiar road, one we traveled together many times when my sons were younger, my parents in their car, my family in ours. This trip, just the three of us, hearkened back even further, to the vacations of my childhood when my parents, my sister, and I went year after year to a little cabin in a tiny Colorado town called Green Mountain Falls. A familiar road but different every time. I wondered what new memories this trip would give us.

The first day was long. We laughed our way through the fields of north Texas, watched the clouds gather and advance from the Oklahoma border, and marveled at the power of the locomotives pulling their steely loads east. By the time we reached the plains of the Texas Panhandle, conversation had slowed and the car was quiet.

I gave thanks for the opportunity to visit these high, arid plains in silence. The trip from Amarillo to Dumas is one of my favorite stretches of highway—anywhere. I reacquainted myself with the vast, stoic expanse. Dry creek beds like wrinkles cutting through the old land, gray with sage and age and cactus that wanted to bloom one more time before winter. Unforgiving land; unapologetic. Proud and quiet. Unafraid of dark and storm and cold. Independent. Promising only to outlive those who crossed over it.

When we reached the motel in Raton, New Mexico, Mom insisted we take everything inside. Not just the luggage, but the maps and the flashlight, all the tools and the battery jumper cables.

"She's tired," Dad said. He didn't let her bring in the floor mats.

I turned on the TV and while Mom watched the news, Dad and I walked to the neighboring café and got hamburgers to carry back to the room. I kept the first twinges of worry to myself.

Later as I prepared for bed, I remembered childhood nights spent in these "little houses," as my sister and I called them. Mom always insisted on scouring the bathroom herself before we were allowed to use it. Her worry over germs made for harrowing moments for two little girls who had already been "holding it" for a long while. I smiled now, thinking of my mother's stubborn overprotective streak.

During the night, I heard her ask my father, "Where are we, Daddy?" She asked the same question again in the early-morning light. As we got out of bed, he told her where the bathroom was— twice. I pushed away my own questions and the worries churning in my mind, even when Mom seemed completely unable to choose what to wear. I suggested the navy slacks and—oh my!— where did she get this great striped blouse? I forced smiles, then felt them for real as I anticipated our visit with Mark.

Finally we all walked to the café where Mom seemed to relax a bit over breakfast. She sat while we repacked the car—when had she become so inactive?—and then we headed north for the last few hours of our trip.

As we drove, I made constant conversation to quell my growing fears. I wondered if Dad was worried. He didn't appear to be, but in most ways, I didn't know him well. He had been the man of the house, taken care of by my mother and revered by my sister and me. He was the father who could build anything, grow anything, repair anything. I watched him do everything my mother asked. He didn't dance, but he loved to sing and did it well. His own father died when Dad was just sixteen, so he left high school to support his mother, brothers, and sisters during the Great Depression. He loved my mother; everyone knew that. But beyond those facts, I could not say I knew my father. Certainly not like I knew Mom and, of course, not like she knew him. For fifty years, she had been reading his moods, speaking his thoughts, and ironing his shirts. It struck me that I hadn't seen her ironing in a long time.

The land stretched to the east in shadowless plains of grass. Rolling, unbroken by hill or tree or house. To the west, the earth erupted in rocky outcroppings, jagged-edged plateaus, and mountains that would soon wear the snow like a comfortable shawl. We drove between them, the grass and the rocks, the gentle flat and the rising sharpness, the sunny plains and the clouded peaks. I sat in the back seat and leaned forward over the console. Dad drove on one side of me and Mom dozed on the other as I sat in the middle and tried to take it all in.

About noon, we turned into the parking lot of Mark's apartment. Mom woke as we parked.

"We're here!" I sang out to her.

"Where?" she growled. "Where are we?"

The next hours remain a vivid nightmare. I have tried in vain to erase the memory of Mom's complete ignorance of where we were and why we had come. Her unbending insistence that we go home immediately. The frantic events of the afternoon. My shock and panic at being powerless to get through to her. And Dad's face, only weary, not surprised.

Mark was still at work. We parked the car outside the door to his apartment, under the outermost branches of a pine tree. Snuggled against the trunk of the tree were two chairs with white paint weathered in spots down to the gray wood. Between them a large, whitewashed pot overflowed with red geraniums.

Somehow we persuaded Mom to get out of the car and go inside. This time she said nothing about all the things we left in the car. We left everything: suitcases packed with clothes for three or four days of sightseeing, hiking boots and walking shoes, an icebox filled with the makings of Mark's favorite dishes. All were left outside while we sat in Mark's apartment awaiting his homecoming.

My mother perched awkwardly on the brown sofa, sitting as though she might spring forward any second. She didn't appear to notice the green and ivory afghan draped across the back and over the arm of the couch, something she would have admired and commented on once upon a time. Dad sat in the only other chair in the little living room, a brown leather recliner given to Mark by an old boss back in Texas. The leather was well worn when it was bequeathed to Mark; it suffered more wear and tear during years of dormitory living and many moves. But now an Indian print blanket covered the back and seat, hiding much of the damage wrought by age and use.

"Is that a television?" Mom pointed to the TV sitting on a table across from the sofa. Framed pictures of family and college buddies covered the edges of the table.

"Yes," I answered. "Would you like me to turn it on?"

"Yeah." Her one-syllable order was low-pitched, surly. As the room filled with noise, Dad stood and walked a few steps to the kitchen, then came back out, walked a step or two into the hall, and looked into the tiny bathroom.

I met him in one of the bedrooms and stated the obvious: "I guess we better get back home."

Before he could speak, Mom's raucous shout rose above the TV chatter. "Where are you two? What are you doing? What are you talking about? Come back in here!"

We obeyed. We hushed. Dad seemed unable or unwilling to discuss the situation.

The hours passed, punctuated every few minutes by Mom's angry questions about where we were and when we were going home. Sometimes Dad answered; sometimes I did. Regardless, the answer was the same.

"We're at Mark's house in Colorado. We'll go home soon."

Finally she simply sat and stared at the television, her furious silence broken occasionally by her muttering to herself, or to the TV advertisers, or to the characters who told cold jokes and laughed hollow laughter into the room. But even after she stopped asking, Dad kept explaining, trying to make her understand. She ignored him and after a while, he gave up. Instead he wandered the rooms with his hands in his pockets jingling his change, stopping to stare out the window toward the chairs arranged so invitingly under the tree. When Mom ordered him to sit down and cut out that infernal noise, he took his hands from his pockets, crossed his arms, and kept walking.

Afternoon became evening and my panic gradually subsided. A

clear-headed, rational anxiety took its place. Was this some extreme temper tantrum thrown by a woman notorious for her willfulness? Was she pretending? Feigning confusion to get the attention she had always craved? I wondered how Mark would react to walking in on such a bizarre situation.

As dusk fell, I decided this must be one of Mark's longer-than-usual workdays. I attempted again without success to get some one of us to eat something. And then while Dad wandered the bedrooms again, Mom announced she was going out for a walk.

"Good idea!" I said. "I'd love a walk!"

No, she was going alone.

"Okay," I agreed, thinking I would follow her at a distance.

I handed her the shoes she'd taken off hours ago. She ignored me and kept walking to the door.

"Mama, you can't go out there barefoot," I said, in as even a tone as I could manage. "It's getting dark. There might be glass in the parking lot."

Still she ignored me. She had made it almost to the door.

"No, Mama!" This time my voice was loud and curt. "You have to wear your shoes." I had never in my life spoken to her that way, never given her an order.

Mom stopped and faced me. Her eyes tightened into slits and her voice slid low as she spoke through gritted teeth. "I'm not putting on any shoes."

I was standing between her and the door when Dad appeared behind her. He's not a large man, but his square frame was a formidable presence looming dark around the edges of her body. He tried for a split second to reason with her, but when she began clawing around me to get to the doorknob, he took her by the shoulders and turned her around. As she struggled to get out of his grasp, he maneuvered her carefully back to the couch. She fell into it, then sat upright, scratching and kicking at him. Making no sound at first, she bared her teeth and thrashed her head to and fro, fighting him with a strength I thought she no longer possessed and the will she had never lacked and would never lose.

I stood rooted to the carpet by the door. Without consciously stringing one thought after another, I arrived at Alzheimer's. I knew symptoms of the disease could fluctuate, especially in the beginning stages; people with the disease could have better times and worse times. I knew that during the bad times, they may not recognize someone as familiar as a daughter or a husband. And I was sure, as I watched the surreal scene of my mother hitting my father's shoulders and kicking his stomach, she didn't realize who he was.

At last I moved, rushing to the couch crying, "Mama! Stop! That's Daddy! It's Daddy! You don't want to hurt Daddy!"

Her eyes still narrow and mean, her foot slicing the air, she shouted, "Yes, I do!"

I can't believe the neighbors didn't bang on the walls to complain. The shouts—his, hers, ours—beat against my ears. Dad's voice boomed louder and louder, "Marie! Marie!" fighting to be heard over her wordless cries of rage.

I guess Mom finally wore herself out. I'm sure nothing I said had any effect on her. As I look back now, I feel certain she did know my father after all, and she knew me. She knew she was angry with both of us. What really happened in that time at Mark's apartment is that *she* began to be unrecognizable to *me*.

That's how I met the disease that came to live with my parents while I was selling software. It had moved in on their lives with slow but steady stealth over the span of four or five years. But there in my son's first apartment, in the splendor of the Rocky Mountains, it introduced itself to me—a cold and cunning beast, arrogant, cruel, feasting on my mother's paranoia, her panic and confusion, her utter lack of judgment, her irrational reaction to being told no. I wanted to fight but had nothing to punch.

Evening became a cold autumn night. And as darkness advanced outside, inside the apartment, by the miracle that in coming years would bless us each time we reached the limits of our endurance, the disease slunk away for a while. It left Mom an empty shell, silent, motionless, until she laid her head on the arm of the couch and I gently covered her with the green and ivory afghan.

When Mark finally came in from work that night, his grandmother greeted him by name. He walked into the little living room and brought with him the fresh air of pure, unknowing happiness. Joy suffused his face to see me and his grandparents in his home. The same joy shone back at him from his grandmother's soft, wrinkled features. As though the last few hours were a bad dream from which she had awakened, one she didn't even remember, Mom accepted Mark's hug and kiss, calling him by name again and again. Dad and I watched, I in utter disbelief, and he with a look that told me: "I've seen this before. Let's just pretend it never happened."

So we did. We ordered in some food and while Mark entertained us with stories of the job that took him to remote areas of mountain wilderness, I thanked the Lord for the wonder of hearing my child describe doing work he had studied for and dreamed of. I thanked God also for the relaxed look of pride and love on Mom's face as she listened, her hand idly patting Mark's arm. Aside from some vagueness in her conversation and mostly inconsequential confusion, nothing in her behavior that night gave any hint of the angry chaos we experienced earlier.

I told Mark about it after my parents had gone to bed. In the deserted laundry room of his complex in the darkest hours of the night, I leaned against the coin-operated dryer and faced him. As the washer churned his flannel shirts and beat against his jeans, I described the nightmare we lived while we waited for him to come home. I couldn't hold back my tears, but I tried to hide what by then had become my utter despair. He cried too, with no sound and no movement. Mark is big and solid as a mountain, tall and straight as a pine, but his heart is tender and his emotions run just under the surface, like a mountain stream rushing hard and fast beneath a thin clear layer of ice. As we stood by the dryer with his arm around my shoulders, I felt him growing older and I cried some more.

The next morning, Dad and I greeted each other with the same conviction—we must go home immediately. Mom asked questions about whose house we were in, where her things were, where to find the bathroom. Dad answered in a tired, sad voice.

9

Finally she asked him, "What's wrong, Daddy?"

"Well, we were going to stay here and visit with Mark for a day or two," he told her. "But you said yesterday you don't want to be here. You want to go home."

"Do you want to stay?" she asked him, looking for all the world like a child preparing a surprise for her parent.

"Yes, but not if you want to go home."

"Then let's just stay." Her voice was triumphant. "If you want to, I do, too!"

So we stayed for just that one day. We walked in the mountains, drove up the river road, and ate pizza at Beau Jo's. Some instinct told me to keep Mom awake and alert as we drove, so I maintained a continuous chatter to her, pointing to the fading blooms of miner's candles beside the road, marveling at the pine, fir, and juniper, twisted and gnarled, struggling to escape skyward from among the boulders that imprisoned their roots.

We stopped occasionally and walked a bit, Dad and Mark tramping ahead with boundless vigor and an unmistakable mutual admiration that brought tears to my eyes. I hung back with Mom, walking slowly, resting often. Much of our talk consisted of one of us saying, "Oh look! Isn't that beautiful?" to which the other would reply, "Oh, yes! It's lovely!" That seemed to be the full extent of her conversational ability, at least while she was walking, but she seemed genuinely happy and I joined in her pleasure.

The only difficult part of that day occurred during one of the visits Mom and I made to bathrooms at our various stops. From outside the stall, I could tell she was using copious amounts of toilet paper. When I asked if she needed help, she opened the door and said, "Yes, please." She had soiled herself. I made light of it, disguising my dismay in order not to embarrass her, and helped her clean herself. What struck me even more than the shock of her "accident" was that I needn't have worried about her embarrassment. She was like a child who felt she'd done nothing wrong, who knew she could rely on me to make things right. It was supremely important to me that no hint of the event reach Mark, but I half expected Mom to tell him and Dad herself. She didn't. I pretended all was well. For Mom, no pretending was needed.

The next morning, we knew with certainty it was time to head back to Texas. The excruciating tension erupted almost as soon as Mom awakened. By the time we loaded the car, she would scarcely tell Mark good-bye. She wasn't speaking at all to me or Dad.

We made the sixteen-hour drive home in fourteen hours. I drove the whole way, very fast, stopping only for gasoline, snacks, a bathroom. At first, Dad and I managed to speak with mock cheerfulness over the nonstop tirade from the back seat. I prayed when Mom's anger boiled over into ranting and shouting; I worried only slightly less when the noise from the back seat stopped entirely. I drove and drove, mile after mile, hanging by a thread that was stronger than I knew. In times to come as I cared for Mom, I would see, not a mere thread, but a bright golden cord twined of hope and help and daily miracles.

Sometime after midnight, we parked in the garage at my parents' house. Over her protests, I helped Mom inside.

"Finally!" she growled. "I thought you'd never find a bathroom!"

We had made it home. And our journey into the heart of Alzheimer's had begun.

NOTES

- Even if you are close to someone with Alzheimer's, the first signs of the disease may be hidden from you.
- The first hints that a loved one has Alzheimer's are sometimes revealed in the changed behavior of a spouse or friend who is trying to adjust to your loved one's new moods and actions.
- Confusion and forgetfulness are not always the first symptoms of Alzheimer's. Abrupt mood changes, hostile behavior, physical aggression, reluctance to drive or go out alone, unreasonable fear, lack of interest in personal hygiene, occasional incontinence, language difficulties, the same questions repeated again and again—these are some of the many other signs that might signal the disease.

> Any of the symptoms associated with Alzheimer's may be caused instead, or also, by other ailments or conditions. That's why it is critically important to acknowledge difficulties like incontinence, confusion, language difficulties and the rest, and call them to the attention of a primary care physician in a timely manner. Don't assume your loved one's physician is already aware of such changes.

> Changes in behavior may be subtle at times, like the inability to order from a restaurant menu, and dramatic at other times, like emotional outbursts or physical aggression.

> Symptoms may be very problematic one day and gone the next, especially in the earliest stages of Alzheimer's.

> My mother's confusion was greater when she awakened in the morning or after a nap during the day. Especially in the beginning, keeping her alert during the day and involved in the activity of the moment seemed to make her feel more secure and greatly increased the likelihood she would eat at meals, accept help with dressing and, in general, work with us instead of against us.

> While it's difficult to predict with certainty what will cause distress to an individual Alzheimer's patient, even early on you will see that certain activities and situations tend to provoke symptoms. Situations like going to an unfamiliar place or being in the company of strangers or in a crowded room were triggers for Mom.

> Once Mom was in an emotional state, trying to reason with her was useless. The best strategy was to agree with her statements and desires as far as possible. For example, it was fine for Mom to go for a walk in a strange place as long as she would wear shoes and as long as I went, seen or unseen, with her.

> But if there is no way to accommodate your loved one's desires, or no way to accommodate them safely, you'll need to be prepared to take the action necessary to keep her safe. I had to exert physical pressure on Mom only one other time after the incident described in this chapter. But if you feel you would be unable to physically restrain your loved one if it became necessary, it's best to have a plan in place. Have a neighbor, friend, or family member you can call for immediate help, or, if all else fails, be prepared to call the police

for assistance. Perhaps such a situation will never arise, but you'll be able to care for your loved one with more confidence and calm if you have faced the possibility in advance and are prepared either to take action yourself or to get help.

Dodging the Bullet

Son of man, look carefully and listen closely and pay
attention to everything I am going to show you, for
that is why you have been brought here.
—EZEKIEL 40:4, NIV

lzheimer's dropped into my life like a roof collapsing on my head. While I recovered from the blow, I tried to keep living as though having no roof were only a minor inconvenience.

"Fix it!" my brain commanded. "Just fix it! It isn't Alzheimer's. It's something else. Something fixable. Like any other illness. Get your mother to a doctor and fix it!"

But my heart didn't believe my brain. Having no roof meant having no place to hide from the harsh reality of Mom's behavior. Yes, she was always a willful woman. She was a strict disciplinarian, first with me and my sister, and then with her grandchildren. She was inclined to think other people didn't like her. She was moody, defensive, secretive. And as she passed into and beyond middle age, these characteristics became more pronounced.

Still, the scenes I witnessed in Colorado went far beyond the actions of someone with a "difficult" personality. As I replayed the trip in my mind, with roof debris around my feet, I was forced to acknowledge the other extreme behaviors Dad and I had been ignoring for the last couple of years.

For instance, Mom went to the same hairstylist for well over thirty years. Ima Jean. Most women will tell you that finding a good hairstylist is as important as finding the right doctor. Knowledge and experience in his or her specialty is important, of course, but it's not enough. Not nearly. Like your doctor, the person who does your hair has to know things about you: your beauty history, the idiosyncrasies of your hair, your taste, what you can tolerate, where you've been in life and where you're going. Ima Jean knew these things about my mother. She was the surgeon who cut off Mom's silky waves when I was in grade school, the healer who cured her indecision about passing beauty fads and treated the dreaded gray. And Ima Jean was a family doctor—err, beautician. She did my hair for proms and later for my wedding. She knew my children. My oldest son used to toddle off to the beauty shop once a week with my mom. Fridays. Every Friday. Doctors came and went. Ima Jean remained. That's how it was. Until the Beauty Shop Battles.

The Battles began three or four years before the fateful Colorado trip, at about the time my mother stopped driving. No real reason for the driving decision; just one day she was afraid to and then one day became every day. So Dad started chauffeuring her on errands and taking her to her hair appointments. Soon the appointments were no longer scheduled for every single Friday; in fact, Dad had a hard time determining any schedule at all for beauty shop days. I knew this because occasionally I visited them on a day when they were discussing my mother's hygiene, which, like the beauty shop appointments and her driving, was falling mysteriously by the wayside. She bathed only when he insisted and then resolutely denied that shampooing was part of bathing.

"But, baby, I wash my hair every time I shower," Dad reminded her.

"Well, I don't. And my hair is fine."

I could have told him that the more he suggested she needed to do a thing, the less likely she was to do it. After fifty years of marriage, how could he not know that? His naiveté in dealing with my stubborn mother never ceased to amaze me.

So there they would sit, across from each other at the breakfast table, Mom glaring at almost-bald Dad from beneath her oily gray-brown hair.

"Okay, baby. No shampoo," he would sigh.

When I was there I kept my mouth shut.

That's how it was during the months just before the trip— Mom's hair receiving little attention until it grew so long it bothered her. She'd worn it short since she was in her mid-thirties; now she couldn't bear the feel of it brushing against her neck. When it reached that point, she would telephone Ima Jean. I was there sometimes when she called. With urgency in every word, she begged for an appointment as soon as possible. Generally she got one within twenty-four hours. But, although Dad always reminded Mom to call him when she was ready to come home, Mom never called. Ima Jean did.

The random routine worked fine for a while. Dad first began suspecting trouble when he noticed the appointments were lasting much longer than the usual forty-five minutes. Sometimes, he said, he waited two and a half or three hours for the call that Mom was ready.

Then came the day Mom fumed about her longtime friend Ima Jean all the way home from the beauty shop. "Ima Jean did two other women's hair before she did mine. I guess she's mad at me. I don't even know who those women were. She likes them better than me."

"Oh, no, baby, that can't be right," my father soothed.

Mom erupted. "Are you saying I'm lying? That's what Ima Jean said. She said I'm a liar. She said I didn't even have an appointment."

As I listened to Dad's story a couple of days later, my mind shifted to silent alarm mode.

"Whoa…what did you say, Daddy?" I asked him.

"What could I say?" He didn't sound alarmed, merely miserable. "Your mother said she made the appointment. But sometimes she forgets things."

Weeks passed and Dad described similar scenarios. Then came the Colorado trip and the secure roof of our lives no longer sheltered us from such incidents. A hot glare illuminated every strange feature of Mom's actions. Try as we might, we could not continue to pretend everything was normal.

The Beauty Shop Battles began again shortly after our return from Colorado. This time, I was there to watch the action. Coming for an afternoon visit, I walked in on a tense moment as Dad questioned whether Mom had really made the phone call for a hair appointment during the short time he was outside collecting mail. The blinds at the breakfast room window were closed to the late-afternoon sun. A cigarette smoldered in my mother's favorite green ashtray; the air was saturated with smoke.

I got something cold to drink and sat down at the table with them as Dad repeated his question.

"Are you sure, baby? You talked to Ima Jean? You really do have an appointment tomorrow?"

The corners of my mother's mouth spread side to side, pulling her lips into a tight line. Slowly she reached toward the ashtray and picked up the cigarette with its long dangling ash. With her elbow planted on the table, she held the unfiltered stub between index finger and thumb. Her eyes were afire through the hanging smoke, staring silent and seething at Dad.

Then *whap!* Her other hand slammed palm down on the table. The ice rattled in my glass; the fire fell from the cigarette and landed on the tablecloth. Instinctively my father reached over and put it out with his hand.

"*Oh my....Marie!* You scared me to death!" He knew better than to shout, but his anger raised the tone of his voice by at least an octave. "What on earth is it?"

"Oh, the big man!" Mom intoned. "The big man wants to know what's wrong. Stop talking! Stop talking about me and Ima Jean! I'm never going back to Ima Jean. Never!" She slammed her hand on the table again.

Dad glared back, his face a mirror of hers. Angry lines cut it into small triangles of eyes and a larger one holding his clenched jaws and chin. But in the long-accepted pattern of their relationship, he said nothing. Nothing about the appointment, nothing about her anger or his, nothing about the newest hole in the tablecloth or the red blister at the base of his thumb. He just turned on the television. The weatherman filled the silence.

Until that day, Mom hadn't staged an outburst nearly as severe as the one that took place in Mark's apartment. Not to my knowledge, at least. But the hand-slamming incident confirmed my fears that her irrational behavior would be repeated. Once again I watched Dad close his eyes to it, in the same way he had kept his mouth closed when I tried to bring up the events of our trip. Dad didn't want to discuss Mom's actions. And up to this point, I had been complicit in his denial. But now I could imagine the table ablaze with a fire started by her cigarette; I could picture her deciding to walk alone out of the house; I saw her slamming her hand against my father instead of the table.

On my next visit a few days later, I spoke to Dad about my fears. While Mom and Charley, their poodle, were watching *Wheel of Fortune*, Dad went outside to check the antifreeze in the cars. I followed him into the garage where I told him that the recent argument at the breakfast table was too close to the explosive behavior Mom had exhibited on the trip.

"I'm worried she might hurt herself when she loses it like that, Daddy. She could hurt you, too."

"No, no, honey." He shook his head and leaned against the hood of his beloved brown pickup truck.

Motor oil, grass shavings on the lawnmower, lawn fertilizer— the garage smells were sweet to me, reminding me of the days when my sister and I played house in here beside my father's tools. She was only sixteen months older than I, but even that small amount of seniority gave her the privilege of choosing to be the mom. I had to be the daddy. I didn't mind.

"You're worrying too much," Dad continued. "I know your mother's ornery sometimes; too much of the time, in fact. She stays mad so much of the time, sometimes I wonder if she's depressed. But she wouldn't ever hurt me. And I promise you I watch that cigarette-smoking every minute."

Sighing, I wondered how he was watching it right this minute, but I didn't call him on it.

"But what if she didn't have to be mad all the time, Daddy?" I asked. "There are so many things that help depression. What if she could feel better? Don't you think it's worth checking into?"

"Oh, I don't know…" His voice trailed off like the wheeze of a tired engine. "Just getting her to go get her blood pressure checked is terrible sometimes."

I took the opening. "We could go and just talk to the doctor, Daddy. You and I could go and tell him what's going on. See what he thinks. Maybe he'll prescribe something the next time she has an appointment."

It took weeks to persuade him. I thought hope would motivate my father, but until he acknowledged the reality of the problem, he had no need for hope. Desperation, finally, was the motivator. The bad times of day began to outnumber the good times, and the difficult days outnumbered the easy ones. On their almost-daily trips to the neighborhood discount store, Mom's penchant for steering a shopping cart into the side of other shoppers' carts helped make my argument. Her refusal to bathe helped too, I think. But her growing habit of cursing at him was the last straw.

Though Dad had cursed on a few dire occasions in my childhood, I never once heard Mom do it. Now she cursed often, and always at my father. I don't believe in their fifty years of marriage he'd ever had a reason to doubt her devotion to him. Until now. When she swore at him, the look on his face told me he was desperate to reclaim her love. He had to prove to himself it lived as always at the heart of the pink brick home that was the center of their now very small world.

Dad had given up vacations; being anywhere other than home with Mom was too difficult. He had let go of their partnership in landscape and home-improvement projects and picked up each task of homemaking as she dropped them one by one. He had even given up much of their conversation as she grew angry with him more and more often. He could not bear to lose more—perhaps couldn't imagine, as she cursed at him, that there was anything more to be lost.

And now Dad knew I had seen the truth. Pretending, to himself and the world, that everything was normal wasn't possible anymore. So finally he agreed to say out loud to the doctor all the things he was living with. I was prepared to add all I had observed. We both knew the speaking would make everything real.

I made the appointment for us to talk to their general practitioner. That day was the second to last time we left Mom at home alone.

The doctor's practice was limited to geriatric care. Dad and the doctor and I sat in a room with an empty examining table. While the doctor took brief notes, Dad and I told him about Mom's behavior during the trip to Colorado. Dad went on to describe her tendency to erupt loudly and physically as she had when discussing her hair appointment. He talked about her rudeness to people in the grocery store and the bizarre stories she told him. He talked about incidents I knew nothing of, including her fear that he had not paid the bills or that the children next door were peeking in the windows.

"I know she's angry, Doctor," Dad finished. "She's sad. I really think depression is making her act this way. I don't know whether anything can be done about that..."

Dad leaned forward in the chair, one arm stretched out, his hand hanging down over his knee. Watching him, I thought of all the meetings he had led in his career, making presentations designed to win business contracts. Surely he had never looked so helpless in a meeting before.

The doctor sat with his head down, taking notes, nodding occasionally. When he looked up, his face was a murky pool. He offered no thoughts, expressed no concern, simply told us to make an appointment and bring Mom in. We agreed.

She didn't.

"Why do I have to go?" she demanded on the designated day. An empty juice glass and half a cup of tepid tea sat before her on the table.

Looking back now, I'm surprised Dad didn't explain all our concerns, assuming she could understand as she would have, say, five years before: "Well you know, honey, you've been so angry lately, and sad. Maybe you're depressed. I'm worried it could even be Alzheimer's. I don't think so, but we do need to get things checked out so you can feel better...".

But he said none of that. He looked at me instead.

"He just wants to look you over, Mama," I said. "A checkup. You know."

"Well, let him look you over," she sneered. Her mood, not good to begin with, deteriorated quickly. "I'm not going."

"Why not, Mama?" I tried to sound calm.

"Because I don't *want* to." She rocked back and forth in her chair.

We dropped the subject for a while. Minutes ticked by. I bit my tongue to keep from talking about a bath. I abandoned any thought of washing her hair and even vowed not to worry about her clothes if only she would agree to go. I prayed silently as Mom kept rocking and the TV newsman droned on about crime and traffic and inclement weather.

When Dad finally spoke, his voice was light. Casual. "Let's go see the ole' doc and then we'll go out for breakfast."

"Oh, Daddy, let's just go to breakfast." Mom smiled at my father. Prayers answered: at least a smile. "I don't need to see the doctor."

Dad smiled back but said nothing. Time passed. More praying. More persuading. More refusing.

And then, suddenly, she gave in. She just said, "Okay."

A miracle.

We even got there on time—Mom with dirty hair, wearing a blouse she had slept in, smelling strongly of cigarette smoke and slightly of urine. She and I sat in blue padded chairs lined against the wall of the waiting room. While Dad paced in the otherwise empty room, jingling the change in his pocket, Mom looked around as if she'd never been there before.

Now and then she leaned over and whispered random comments in my ear: "Look at that plant." When she pointed, I had to pull my head back to avoid injury.

"I don't like that picture." Last month, she thought it was one of the prettiest pictures she'd ever seen.

"Tell your father to sit down." I ignored that one.

Finally the nurse called her name. As the three of us walked toward the examining room, I realized I was holding my breath.

But why was I worried? There she was, stepping on the scale when she was directed to, gushing a thank you to the nurse who took her blood pressure. Was this Mom? The Mom who was hissing and growling a few hours ago? Where had she been hiding that angelic expression?

Pulse? Temperature? Yes, yes! Thank you! The examining room was cold, but as we waited on straight-backed metal chairs, Mom never complained.

Finally the doctor came in. He was approaching middle age, not tall, but slender, with dark complexion and black hair, straight and thick. Mom greeted him with a wide smile, which he returned, looking, I thought, a bit surprised. They exchanged comments about how nice the weather had been. Then he listened to her heart and lungs.

"No need to get up on the table," he said. "We can do this right here in your chair."

I could read her face. Such a nice man, she was thinking. In the next couple of minutes, he educated her on the value of exercise and she politely agreed to stop smoking.

Then the doctor asked, "Are you depressed, Mrs. Bailey?" His clipped accent made the question sound light and conversational.

"Noooo." She smiled and drew the word out as though she found the question strange and a little funny.

The doctor smiled too, and even chuckled a little as he continued. "You're not worried about anything? Afraid about anything?"

"Oh, no!" Her voice was calm and sincere, and she turned lovingly to Dad. "We're just fine, aren't we, Daddy?"

"You bet, baby!" he boomed in reply. "You and me and Charley-Dog! We're great!"

If my jaw actually dropped as my parents stood to go, no one called it to my attention. Until that moment, I had utterly underestimated the extent of Dad's denial. The growling and shouting that still echoed in my mind, the kicking and the flailing on the couch in Mark's apartment—all was apparently erased from his memory by Mom's look of love and her "We're fine, aren't we, Daddy?"

The doctor smiled and left the room with a cheery, "See you in four months!"

Still in shock, I walked my parents to the car. The anger would hit me later. Anger at the absurdity of the doctor's questions and at Dad's dizzying retreat to denial. Even anger at Mom, though I tried to convince myself she had no control over her sweetness and normalcy before this one man who might have helped us all. But I saved most of the anger for myself. My fear infuriated me.

Yes, of course, I should have told the doctor that this was the sunny side of my mother's behavior, a side we seldom saw anymore. "Company" behavior, the kind she exhibited when we had visitors. But I was afraid to say that in front of her. Scared of what she would do. I thought she'd probably react with the cold hostility she displayed so much of the time at home. But isn't that what we wanted? So the doctor could see that behavior for himself?

No. I was afraid of it. I was terrified that her anger would work itself up into the frenzy we'd seen at Mark's apartment. Could we control her? Would she run? Start thrashing her arms and legs? Break something? Grab the needles, smash the equipment, turn over chairs in the waiting room? Would she hurt herself? Someone else?

Escape was the only option I saw. Escape from the situation without doing anything to provoke the wild woman who lived in my mother's body. So, coward that I was, I kept silent and we walked to the car.

Breakfast after the doctor's visit was quiet but pleasant as Mom's fine mood continued. No one at the small neighborhood restaurant my parents frequented seemed surprised at her appearance.

When we got home, the three of us sat in our customary places around the table. Neither Dad nor I brought up the doctor's visit. I sensed he was as loathe as I to disturb Mom's good cheer. To someone from the outside, our conversation and laughter would indicate we were having a grand time.

The light from the window in the breakfast room grew brighter and warmer as early afternoon became late, then mellowed as evening became night. My parents spent more time at this table now than anywhere else in their home. On the best days, they feasted on their life there, recalling past events, happy or sad, dreaming of a future that was bright and expansive, though their vision of it stretched only a few days forward. And this had been a good day. After a difficult start, it had grown fat and happy with the doctor's implied diagnosis: nothing wrong here.

An observer would never guess that Dad and I were hostages, held captive by Mom's moods and outbursts. For now though, the outbursts were only bad memories. Today we had dodged the bullet of our worst fear: the word *Alzheimer's*. Dad and I both thought it occasionally, but neither of us wanted to hear a doctor put that name to Mom's malady. Until a doctor said it, we didn't have to believe it.

NOTES

> For me, one of the first and most difficult challenges of living with someone with Alzheimer's was determining when Mom was speaking about reality and when she was speaking out of her confusion. Eventually Dad and I learned to treat everything Mom said as real, since, in her perception, it was real. Arguing with her or trying to persuade her otherwise never worked. At best, it made her more confused; at worst, it made her furious with us. So we acted as though we believed all she said was true. If we needed to double-check—as, for instance, when she said a doctor called and told her an appointment had been cancelled—we did it out of her earshot.

> Smoking and Alzheimer's do not mix. No matter how careful you are, there will be problems, perhaps even life threatening problems, from fallen or dropped cigarettes. (See "Helps" for more information about how we dealt with Mom's smoking.)

> Be aware that your doctor may be inclined, especially at first, to put more weight on what he sees from his patient than on what he hears from you. If you find that's the case, you'll want to be persistent in documenting for him the behavior he doesn't see in his office. You'll need to make yourself heard.

> Even Mom's most irrational behavior and extreme confusion didn't convince my father that he should consider the possibility she had Alzheimer's. Be aware that it might require time and patience to help a loved one accept that diagnosis.

Just a Little Off the Sides

Praise be to the Lord, for he showed me the wonders of his love.... In my alarm I said, "I am cut off from your sight!" Yet you heard my cry for mercy when I called to you for help.
—PSALM 31: 21–22, NIV

Before my mother's next visit with the doctor, I was offered a job. After the trip to Colorado, I had continued to seek new employment, even though I dreaded the thought of telling my father he was on his own again. He was on his own or he could get outside help. I knew that's what I would have to say. But even as I sent out resumes, the words stabbed me. What would they do to Dad?

So while I prepared for interviews, I also rehearsed the speech I would give my father. "Daddy, I have a new job. We must hire someone to help you take care of Mama. You can't go through this alone when I go back to work."

It sounded so reasonable. It *was* reasonable. He'd see that.

Though I spent most afternoons with my parents, I was at home on the early spring afternoon when the job offer came. The phone call interrupted my cleaning a closet. Wrapping paper of every color and pattern had been spread across the floor as I emptied the shelves. Gift bags, tissue paper, ribbon, padded mailing envelopes, foam peanuts, packing tape: everything one could ever need to wrap a gift and send it near or far was now restacked in the closet.

I craved order and cleanliness, wherever I could find them or impose them, so it had been a bright, satisfying afternoon. I had only to bag up the discards and carry them out to the garbage when the telephone rang.

The offer was good. I was well qualified for the job. The salary was within the range I had set during the interviews.

"I can let you know in a couple of days. By Friday. Thank you so much."

I hung up the telephone and felt physically ill. I couldn't stop inhaling. The afternoon closed in around me and the air which before had been warm was now hot and thick. I sat on the floor beside the closet debris, held my head in my hands, and wondered what I had done.

How could I leave my father alone with the nightmare he was living? How could I skip off to collect a paycheck as he struggled to get through each day with his sanity intact? Of course it wasn't just the paycheck I wanted; it was the opportunity to do what I was skilled at doing. It was structure in the midst of the chaos that had filtered into every other corner of my life. It was contributing to my own family's well-being, instead of imposing on them the burden of my mother's condition. But I jumped past those benefits and went instead to the questions that screamed in my head. Who else would help my father? Who would help him talk my mother into going to the doctor? Who would read the mail when he was too frustrated to use his magnifying glass? Who would drive them to unfamiliar places? Who but me? Who else?

My sister wasn't a candidate. She and her husband lived just a few blocks from my parents. She had raised six children who now lived close by; she was a loving and involved mother and grandmother. But she did not see my parents' situation as her problem. I believe she would have felt the same even if I hadn't already stepped into the situation with both feet. But after I did, it was mine to deal with.

"I have to work," she told me. "I'll help when I can, but I have to work."

Often in our childhood, in times of my mother's emotional absence or in her too-harsh presence, my sister had taken care of me. But now she had to work. So who else was there?

Sitting on the carpet I had planned to shampoo the next week,

I wept as I had not wept even on the night in Mark's laundry room. Loud, groaning, rocking forward then looking at the ceiling, I cried. Then I prayed. In the suffocating indecision of that hour, I considered no options beyond two: I could take the job and leave my parents alone and desperate—that's how I saw it—or I could refuse the job and join their desperation. So frantic was I for direction, a sign, that I made a bargain with myself: I would call the company back and ask for more money. If they were willing to pay it, I was supposed to take the job. If they declined, I would decline.

By the end of that day, my decision had been made. I didn't consult my husband about it; I simply informed him when he arrived home that night. The company wouldn't pay more so I turned down the job.

"You're handling this like it's a crisis," he told me.

"It is! It is a crisis! If this isn't a crisis, what is?"

"I mean you're treating it like it's a sudden emergency, something you have to move heaven and earth to deal with, but something that will get worked out in a short amount of time. This is going to be a long-term problem for your mom, your father. And for you. For the whole family. You can't just throw yourself at it and expect to resolve it any time soon. We're looking at years!"

His words scarcely registered with me.

Options. Why didn't I see them? I had started walking this steep, rocky path with my father, both of us trying to hold my mother steady as she walked through the rest of her life. Now all I could see was that my stepping off the path would mean disaster for both of them.

So the weeks stumbled by, all of us lurching along through Mom's near-constant hostility. She spoke many times of a man who, she said, had come to the door to tell her that the fence surrounding the backyard was a few inches into the neighbor's property and so the house my parents had lived in for forty years would be repossessed. She asked repeatedly whether a certain bill had been paid. When she was in the car with us, she shouted at people in other cars. At home, she argued with advertisers and newscasters on TV. She continued bumping her cart into others at the grocery store and occasionally made faces at children.

27

Worst of all for Dad and me to bear were the days Mom spent wishing she were dead. Sitting on her green velvet couch with Charley-Dog at her side, she stared across the room at the venetian blinds which she insisted must be kept closed. Brown curtains saturated with years of cigarette smoke were an additional barrier to the light and life going on outside.

"I just wish I could die. I wish I could die," she said through clenched teeth. From the table where Dad and I sat, he struggled to get to make her hear him. Approaching her physically when she was in this state of mind usually made things worse, so he spoke his heart long distance, from the round bright spot where he wanted her to be to the dark dingy rectangle where she sat.

"No, no, baby. Don't say that, baby. You don't want to die and leave me here alone, do you? Don't you love me?"

No, she didn't love him; she didn't care if she left him alone. She just wanted to die. She didn't care about anyone or anything. She wanted to die.

I said nothing at those times. Why? Partly because I didn't trust Mom. I wasn't certain she meant it. Perhaps she was manipulating us to get her way. It wouldn't be the first time.

During the period of Mom's illness when she vacillated so radically, seeming lucid and "with us" for part of the day and so far from rational at other times of the day, I frequently found myself furious with her. I doubted her illness. It seemed as if she knew she had the power to cause pain and chaos. As if she were choosing to be hurtful, not just to me, but to this man who did everything for her. Expressing anger did not come easily for me in any event, but certainly not to my mother, and certainly not in this situation where, as I tried so hard to convince myself, *She can't help it. She's sick. She can't help it.* So I stayed silent.

We didn't wait for the four months to pass before we returned to the doctor's office. Dad and I went again without Mom. As we had done the time before, we gave the doctor written descriptions of her behavior. He could read them at his convenience, put them in her file. As before, he scarcely glanced at them.

But this time the doctor did agree to give her some tests when he saw her next. He didn't believe she was depressed. He thought she had some form of old-age dementia.

Dad stopped him at that point.

"Look, Doctor," he said firmly. "I don't want Marie written off to Alzheimer's."

That wouldn't happen, the doctor assured us.

"Alzheimer's," he told us, "is a gut-wrenching diagnosis for any physician to make."

Persuading Mom to come with us on the appointed day was as difficult as before. We had expected the struggle; this time we dared not hope for the miraculous resolution we had experienced last time.

"No!" she shouted. "I am not going to see any doctor!!"

Then she stood, turned, and in a flash picked up the dining chair where she'd been sitting. She who at times could scarcely raise a fork to her mouth lifted the chair higher, over her head, repeating "No! No! No!" in a throaty growl.

Though I was standing next to Mom, her next actions caught me completely off guard. Before I could reach around the dried-up sapling shape of her body, she stepped back, opened her fingers, and with a flourish let her hands fly out to the sides. The chair hit the floor, seeming to crash separately on each of its four legs.

Standing with her arms over her head like a winning prizefighter in the center of the ring, Mom smiled a wide, cold smile. Then, either not noticing or not caring that it now faced the back of the room, she sat back down in the chair.

Neither my father nor I spoke. What words made any sense in that moment? What response made even a glimmer of sense? We just looked at each other. Even Dad's eyes said nothing.

As I watched the hands of the kitchen clock turn, my mind dredged up a scene from many years past: me, sitting at the bedside of my father-in-law as he lay dying. The glowing red numbers of the digital clock in his darkened room flipped dramatically as each minute passed. I remembered counting his irregular breaths while I waited for the heavy turn of each moment. But here, now, there was no distraction, no escape. Staring at the walls, the clock, the floor, Mom's feet—I wished for something, anything, to count.

An hour or so later, I realized the silence seemed…what? Friendlier. Mom had turned in her chair. The chair itself still faced the wall, but she sat sideways in it now. As Dad was leafing through a seed catalogue, she leaned over the table, stretching to see the pictures of "exceptional red globe radishes," so big and bright they were sure be "the envy of all the other gardeners in the neighborhood." Dad loved radishes. Radishes and onions: able to survive the last cold spells of an early Texas spring, when he could no longer withstand the urge to plant something.

"What are those, Daddy?" Mom asked.

Had she forgotten her earlier tirade or was this her effort to start over?

"Radishes, baby!" As though he'd been holding his breath, Dad's response sprang out like a little explosion of relief. "Hey," he continued, stretching across the table toward Mom and whispering dramatically. "Don't you think you better ask Katrinka to help you with your shoes? Then I'll walk you out to the car!"

"Where are we going?" She still leaned toward him, smiling.

"You know, baby! We're going to see the doctor and then get something to eat."

I was bending at Mom's feet, shoes in hand. I prayed as I waited to hear what she'd say.

"Oh! Okay, Daddy."

It worked.

Nothing different. Nothing added or subtracted. Just doing what had worked for us before: mention the doctor's visit as if it were the thing we had planned and looked forward to all morning. Wait a while, try again. The strategy worked.

Again without bathing, with dirty hair and rumpled clothes, Mom walked into the doctor's office and smiled. Again she was polite and pleasant with him. She agreed again to stop smoking, and again she said she was not unhappy.

But this time there were questions. The tests the doctor had spoken of were not lab tests. They were mental exams, conducted orally. From my seat in the corner, I looked at the small-framed elderly woman who was my mother, dressed in her favorite green sweater and her spotted black slacks, silhouetted against the medicine gray of the examining room walls. When the doctor announced he was going to ask her some questions, she nodded slightly. Did I imagine the look of panic in her eyes? I doubt it. My heart ached for her.

When the doctor asked, "Mrs. Bailey, are you unhappy? Are you depressed?" she said, "No" as she had on that last visit. But this time, she was looking at my father with uplifted eyebrows and an expectant smile. "Is that right, Daddy?"

"I don't know, honey. He's asking you, not me. Just tell him."

"I'm fine." She turned back to the doctor. "I'm just fine."

Then the doctor began the memory questions. I learned later these were standard queries intended to determine the extent, if any, of a patient's memory loss. This was the first time I heard them. Within a year, I would have them memorized. Remember these three words: table, penny, apple. Where are we? What city? What state? Who is the president? What year is this? What month? What day of the week is it? What were those three words?

I don't know if the doctor's guts were wrenching, but mine were. Although she answered two or three of his questions in some sketchy form, Mom's reaction to most of them was to shuffle her feet and rock in her chair. Her mouth would open but no words came out.

Sometimes she said, "Oh, wait just a minute now. I know that." And then—nothing. The silence that followed each query seemed to be pulling the air out of the room. Question after question, each one consumed more of the room's oxygen; I felt myself suffocating.

When Mom looked to Dad, he said nothing. Even turned away. So she turned to me. Certain I would help. Certain. And I would have. If my smiles and heartache could have conveyed the answers to her, she would've made a perfect score on the test.

At last, mercifully, it was over. The doctor looked at Dad and me and said he would write a prescription for Aricept, a drug known to relieve some Alzheimer's symptoms for some people. He told us to come back in three months, then nodded his head and left. Both of us knew.

The "gut-wrenching diagnosis" had been made. In the space of twenty minutes in this little examining room in a small suburban medical suite, a doctor had seen the enemy and named it Alzheimer's. To him it must have appeared a quiet enemy, living in my mother's frail body, smiling out her mouth, lumbering through our lives with clumsy steps and a blank expression. An enemy that killed slowly, inexorably, but without a lot of noise. Though Dad and I knew differently, the doctor didn't wait to hear. He just gave our adversary a name and left.

I was furious. "See you in three months." He had no idea what he was asking us to do. Not a clue.

At the end of that long, frustrating day, we were sure of only one thing: God had gotten us to the doctor's office. After the morning's crashing defeat, neither of us had expected Mom's sudden cooperation. Yet a merciful God used a vegetable catalog to win the victory.

But this time the miracle was bittersweet. I knew it was God's care for Mom and for us, but today his care had led to the diagnosis I feared most. He had led us to the truth, but I felt trapped, not free.

The weeks that staggered by after this visit were different in only one respect. The Aricept, Dad declared through pursed lips, made an excellent laxative. It didn't help Mom's memory and confusion, which was the desired effect, or her mood, which it was never designed to do but which would have been the more important aid by far. All it did was complicate the already immense problem with her personal hygiene.

My mother was a beautiful woman when she and my father married. She loved nice clothes and adored shoes. When my sister and I came along, Mom took up sewing. She made all of our clothes and most of her own. She wore little makeup; lipstick sufficed for all but two or three days of the year. Still she was lovely. But she was never much on bathing. One of eleven children in a Depression-era family, I doubt she took a bath more than once a week when she was growing up. She never adopted the habit of a daily bath or shower.

Perhaps that's the reason we'd been able to ignore the decline in her efforts at personal cleanliness for such a long time. Now, month by month as we waited for the next doctor's appointment, she slowly dropped *all* concern for her looks and hygiene. She wouldn't even wash her hands unless we insisted, and sometimes not then. The length of her hair was the only element of her appearance that bothered her. "I can't stand this mess!" she would say, running fingernails brown with nicotine through the gray-brown strands brushing the top of her collar. "I can't stand it!"

Leaping at the opportunity, we would offer to take her immediately to a hairdresser.

"No, no!" She was insulted. "I can't go to just anyone! What do you think I am? A dog?"

So we would suggest going to Ima Jean. I knew we'd have some explaining to do if we called her. Neither Dad nor I had ever talked to Ima Jean about the last visit Mom made to her shop, although we both knew something was wrong with Mom's version of the events. I don't know whether we were embarrassed or afraid of what we might hear. But Ima Jean would understand. We could schedule the appointment at a time when she had no other clients, and I would go with Mom, stay with her. Everything would be fine.

Of course I didn't say all that to Mom. "Just for a trim," I told her. "It won't take any time at all. I'll take you and go in with you and visit with Ima Jean. I don't know how long it's been since I've seen her!"

But no. Mom had forgotten a lot of things, but her determination that she would "never go to Ima Jean again" remained firmly fixed in her mind. So we waited for the day when she would suddenly say "okay" to dropping in somewhere for a haircut.

Meanwhile, I went to a presentation one evening given at a nearby nursing care facility. A geriatric psychiatrist gave a talk about depression in the elderly population. He explained that the anger and aggression sometimes associated with depression is never normal, not even if someone has a terminal disease. Not even if someone has Alzheimer's. Modern antidepressants, he said, can help to regulate the body's chemistry, sometimes providing dramatic relief of anxiety and hostile behavior.

We made an appointment for Mom with this psychiatrist, but she refused to go. "No doctor but mine!" she screamed again, and this time there was no reprieve.

So again, Dad and I went alone. The doctor was kind. He listened to Dad intently, his eyes never leaving Dad's face. But without Mom there, the psychiatrist could do little. He did suggest the possibility of "Alzheimer's," uttering that word as gently as it could be said. He agreed to see Mom any time we could persuade her to come, and recommended we read a book that would give us insight into Alzheimer's.

The car was silent on the drive home, Dad and I once again lethargic with despair. I pondered the cruel irony: Mom wouldn't go see the doctor who might be of the most help to her, while the doctor she would see offered little hope or help.

As the days and weeks passed, Mom's hair continued to grow and, along with it, our collective frustration. We were all taken prisoner in the Beauty Shop Battles. The early effects of Alzheimer's had led to Mom's refusal to go back to the hairdresser; now the problem with her hair was feeding her black moods, exaggerating the effects of the disease. She became angrier with us, angrier with Ima Jean, angrier with everyone except Charley-Dog, who also needed a bath and a haircut.

So it was appropriate, perhaps, that Charley was the only witness to the last skirmish of the Battles. Mom fought alone. She was enemy and ally, victor and vanquished.

I heard about it after the fact.

On the day after the final battle, I walked into their house in my usual state of mind: worried, weary though the day was still new. I never knew what I would encounter when I walked through the door. But there was Mom, already dressed and drinking her tea— thank goodness!—sitting with Dad at the table. The only surprise this morning was the floppy brown hat sitting on her head. My mother never wore hats.

As I got my own tea and made small talk, she remained quiet. Usually that meant she was angry, but today she didn't seem so. She just sat with a smile that struck me as—what? Sad? I watched Dad watching her. The light words he spoke didn't match the heavy look in his eyes. Something was up. I sat down.

"How do you like your mother's hat, Katrinka?" Dad asked, using the nickname for me that was his alone.

The question shot tension into every corner of the room. "Well, yes!" I looked toward Mom. "That is a surprise this morning!" I had learned to speak to her in few words and simple. When she had to work to understand what I said, she grew anxious.

"Daddy got this for me," she said, reaching up to touch the brim of the hat. She shifted in her chair, almost stood, then sat again.

"Your mother asked me how to cover up her head, so I got her one of my extra hats." His tone made it clear he was about to reveal a secret.

"What happened, Daddy?" Mom asked with a look of confusion that bordered on panic. Apparently she too could read his ominous tone but had forgotten what prompted it.

"What do you mean 'What happened'?" Dad shouted. "Show Katrinka your hair! What's left of it!"

Now she remembered. Sadness wandered across her face and she laid her hand gently on top of the hat. "Oh no, Daddy. No. My hair is ruined."

"I'll say it is!" In his anger, Dad almost came out of his chair. "You cut it all off!"

Like lightning, her anger struck. "Just look, child! Look what Ima Jean did to me!" She lifted the brown cloth hat, held it suspended over her head for a second or two, then pulled it back down almost to her ears. Even in that tiny glimpse I could see the damage. She had not cut her hair; she had chopped it. Hacked it.

As I stared, Mom took off the hat again and threw it across the table. In most places, her hair was about half an inch long. In random patches, tufts of maybe an inch stuck out or cowered against her head. Her scalp was visible in long gashes and at odd angles. There was nothing, no hair at all, around her face— nothing across her forehead, nothing around her ears.

I stood and leaned over her, looking for cuts on her head and neck. I didn't see how she could have gotten the hair so short without catching her scalp in the scissors, but I saw no blood.

Still staring, I sat back down. Finally I realized Dad's words were still bouncing off the walls.

"Ima Jean? It wasn't Ima Jean! It was you! You just wrecked it! You haven't seen Ima Jean in months! You did it! Don't blame it on her! If you'd gone to her when we tried to get you to..." On and on he went.

Later in the day, with some new information from Dad, I tried to make sense of the story.

Mom had been upset about her hair all afternoon the day before. "I have to get this mess cut. Or just let me die."

"Tomorrow, baby," Dad had told her. "We'll get it cut tomorrow. It's too late today."

She had continued the chant after I left, Dad said. He'd gone outside for a while, to water the tomato plants, to fill the birdfeeder, to collect the mail. To escape, I supposed. When he came in a few minutes later, Mom wasn't at the table where he'd left her.

He called her name, then saw the light on in the dressing room, a pretty little room next to her bathroom, cameo pink, with mirrors that curved around to reflect every angle, every view. I could imagine what Dad must have seen, but he told me anyway. A massacre. Hair in chunks and dirty clumps on the dressing table, the carpet, clinging to her clothes. Hair, hair. And Mom, he said, wild with the scissors, grabbing at her head, trying to find more strands to lift up and cut off. Miraculously, neither of them was hurt as Dad disarmed her.

I sat at the table trying to look at Mom's eyes instead of the top of her head. I was mostly unsuccessful. She remained adamant she had not done this to herself. Ima Jean had done it. We explained to her a dozen times in the next two hours that we could not "fix" her hair; it would have to grow out. We went out and bought her a hat of her own, two in fact: one a man's hat she insisted she must have, and the other a little red ball cap my father chose. A couple of days later, she refused to wear either of them. And a couple of days after that, both hats disappeared completely. Many things Mom decided she disliked disappeared completely.

Though it would seem there were no victors in the Beauty Shop Battles, the wonder is that this haircut accomplished what all our meeting with and explaining to and questioning of doctors could not.

The family doctor assigned to my parents at the senior healthcare center had decided—out of a wealth of experience, I'm sure, but experience that did not include living with this patient and her pain and her moods twenty-four hours a day—that my mother had Alzheimer's. He had decided the symptoms he saw in his office were not those of a depressed or anxious woman. And the symptoms he had not yet seen? The ones Dad and I had brought to him verbally and also written in careful detail? He simply didn't consider them.

Until he saw the haircut. About two weeks after the Dressing Room Massacre, Mom's regular doctor's appointment found us once again persuading and prodding her into his office. Once again her demeanor became placid and cooperative as soon as we entered the medical building. Once again Dad and I came armed with written questions and two different descriptions of Mom's anxiety, paranoia, and anger: one version, a list of succinctly stated bullet points; the other, a longer, detailed description of incidents and moods and behaviors. Once again we were prepared to plead for this doctor's help.

We didn't have to say a word. When the doctor walked in and saw Mom's hair, his face registered instant alarm.

He looked at my father and asked, "Did she do this?"

Dad just nodded.

Mom sat smiling while the doctor asked my father questions about her behavior. Dad answered patiently, and when the questions slowed, handed the doctor the sheets of paper we'd brought. Instead of stuffing them into the back of her file as he'd done twice previously, the doctor read them, asking for clarification or more details, taking notes. Then he told us he was prescribing a strong antidepressant. He emphasized it would do nothing to improve her memory or lessen her confusion, but it should relieve her anxiety and brighten her mood somewhat. He went on to explain that a geriatric psychiatrist came to his office once a month; he himself would set up a time for the psychiatrist to see my mother.

The turnaround that took place in the examining room that day was a wonder to experience. After a year of trying to get the doctor's attention—to make him begin to treat my mother, not just the symptoms he witnessed—it was neither I nor my father who made him see the light. It was Mom and her haircut. My mother and what the doctor called "her self-destructive tendencies."

I called it a miracle. Before she ever took one of the little pills that would prove so critically important in improving the quality of her life and ours, I knew it was a miracle that had gotten us to this point. Only a miracle could take the pain and madness of that afternoon in the dressing room and turn it to some healing use.

The Beauty Shop Battles were over. Using heretofore undiscovered skills, I cut Mom's hair from that day on, gently and playfully ambushing her with a burgundy plastic cape and tiny silver hair shears on mellow afternoons as she sat at the table chuckling at Dad's corny jokes. Such afternoons became more plentiful after she began taking the antidepressants.

In addition, the family physician became like a brand new doctor for us. Now he would listen. Now he was on our team. And not only did Mom have a good doctor, she'd also found a new hairstylist.

Life was good.

NOTES

▸ In the beginning of my journey with my parents down the Alzheimer's road, I never considered how long the trip might be. I acted as though every difficult situation we encountered was a crisis—we must solve it, I thought, and then we'll never have to deal with it again. I didn't pace myself. I wasn't prepared, emotionally or physically, for the long-term nature of the illness. If I had been more educated about the disease, I hope I would have taken steps immediately to secure help of some kind for my parents. If not for the present, then for later, when the illness might bring burdens we couldn't bear alone. Education is available, from individuals or through day-long caregiver seminars, in books, on tapes, on the Internet. In my case, by the time I went to a caregivers' seminar, I was so panic-stricken, I wasn't able to take full advantage of what I heard. I urge you to get informed early. Information really is power.

▸ Some of the most important information you need has to do with your options for caring for your loved one. There are options. I never acknowledged that fact. There are options. Believe it early and seek them out.

➤ Depression may sometimes precede or accompany Alzheimer's, but, as the psychiatrist we consulted told us, it is never normal. I urge you—don't hesitate to consult your physician about the possibility your loved one is suffering from depression in addition to Alzheimer's.

➤ My mother was, for as long as I can remember, what I would call a "difficult" person. If your loved one also has a "grumpy" personality, keep in mind that, especially in the early stages of the disease, it may be difficult to distinguish between the unreasonable behavior of a difficult person and the irrational behavior and confusion of someone with Alzheimer's.

Morning Has Broken

This I call to mind and therefore I have hope: because of the Lord's great love we are not consumed, for his compassions never fail. They are new every morning; great is your faithfulness.

—LAMENTATIONS 3:21–23, NIV

Around seven each morning, with the smell of urine strong in his nostrils and a dread of what the day ahead would hold, my father would awaken in the bed he and my mother still shared after fifty-two years. Early in Mom's illness, the bed was sometimes wet; later that was the case most days; eventually, it was every day. But, by some miracle, the dampness was usually confined to her side.

It never occurred to Dad to sleep in another bed. He would have dismissed even the suggestion of it as ridiculous. Wet sheets and foul smells were a depressing wake-up call. They were persistent problems, never satisfactorily solved, but to Dad they were an acceptable price to pay to have Mom still sleeping at his side each night. She was the love of his life, and each morning he confronted the ugliness of Alzheimer's with his steadfast determination to make her day as good as possible.

Mom almost always slept later than Dad, another miracle that preserved some calm for him at the beginning of the day. He rose quickly, quietly. As he dressed, he was watched by two pairs of unblinking eyes that smiled out at him from a large portrait of my sister and me, ages five and four. It had hung on the wall of my parents' bedroom since they bought the house. Forty-three years. When Dad moved to the kitchen to turn on the teakettle, those eyes kept watch as Mom slept on, with Charley-Dog at her feet.

If she stayed asleep long enough, Dad could sit at the kitchen table and enjoy the morning news, relatively stress-free. "Relatively," because even with Mom asleep he was still at the mercy of his own troubling thoughts. What new problems would the day bring? What new losses? Of more immediate importance, what kind of mood would Mom bring to the breakfast table?

Morning and bedtime were the most difficult times of Dad's day. But when he spoke of them, he used only the most general of terms. Detail was lacking in his descriptions because he knew details would give me ammunition. Armed with specific examples of the problems he faced each morning, I could have been specific about the ways a home health care provider could help him.

Even without details, I pressed him to get help.

Same response, every time I brought it up: "I can't do that, baby. How could I schedule someone? I never know whether your mother will sleep until eight o'clock or eleven. What would a helper do? Sit here at the table with me and wait? I won't have that. I'd feel invaded. Besides, I can handle it fine."

"Invaded." The word I heard for years—first with Mom's illness and later with his own—to describe Dad's distaste for having "a stranger" in his home. I wish I had fought harder to show him that the stranger might become a friend.

Instead I became the helper. Once I made up my mind that a full-time job was out of the question for me, I slipped into believing I had to be at my parents' house every day. At first I came around noon. But as I observed more of the overwhelming nature of Mom's needs, I arrived earlier. That's when I began to see the details of Dad's mornings, their mornings, in person.

Mornings began with tea. When my parents were dating in the 1940s, Dad drank only coffee. Mom, whose parents entered the United States through Ellis Island from England, drank only tea. Eventually she learned to *drink* coffee, but she never learned to *make* it. So Dad learned to drink tea. To say he drank it hot is an understatement. He

41

drank it scalding hot, with nothing added. He used the same tea bag to make at least two cups, sometimes three. I, on the other hand, drank tea as my grandmother had taught me: very strong, with sugar and milk. At first Dad was aghast that I used a fresh teabag for every cup. Though delivered with a little smile in a teasing tone, there was no mistaking the pressure of his almost-daily question: "*Another* teabag?" Surprisingly, I didn't acquiesce to his unspoken request. I almost never challenged him, even when I knew he was wrong, wrong to the point of harm to my mother. But when it came to breakfast drinks, I was strong as steel.

That first hour of the day, while Mom was still in bed, grew sweeter as time passed, for both Dad and me. It was a gift, moments when he could keep up with the events of the world outside the pink brick house, and moments when I could watch him, listen to his thoughts about those events, and finally get to know him better.

But while we sipped our tea and watched the news, we listened closely for the jangle of Charley-Dog's collar. The noise meant Charley was awake and probably jumping down from the bed, and that was a pretty reliable signal that Mom was awake, too. We learned to check often to see if she was getting out of bed, so we could intercept her and help her to the bathroom.

As Alzheimer's stole from Mom any notion of personal cleanliness, she never "needed" to go to the bathroom anymore. Disposable underwear was the only solution. But even night-time disposables were often no match for her bladder and bowels, especially after a night of blessedly sound sleep. So Dad and I listened very carefully in the mornings.

Sometimes we didn't hear her soon enough. And sometimes, even when we did hear, things went badly. She was unsteady on her feet when she first arose, so one of us would take her arm and lead her gently toward the bathroom, just around the corner from their bed. A slight turn to the left, and we could help her get clean, dry, and comfortable for the day, or most of it. But too often she insisted on going the opposite way.

"I don't need to go in there," she would say. "I want to go sit down."

With determination born of confusion and fear and long-practiced willfulness, with physical strength she seldom demonstrated except in anger, she would pull away and insist on sitting "There!" on the couch, or "There!" at the kitchen table.

Every inch of her clothing would be soaked, sometimes dripping. With each step, she soiled the wall-to-wall carpet, which covered beautiful wood floors she used to polish on her hands and knees. Reasoning with her was impossible. We would speak lovingly to her. Cajole. Dad would try firmness, even anger. Occasionally she relented. Or maybe she just gave up. But usually if the morning started with her decision for no bathroom and no dry clothes, the passing moments brought no quick relief. We were pretty sure to hear "no" to her medication; "no" to breakfast; "no, you don't" to my father's "I love you"; and an angry "leave me alone" when we tried to help her.

At the point where turning left meant hope and turning right meant misery, Dad could fight her. He could try to hold her still and remove wet clothing from flailing arms and kicking legs. Or he could surrender. He always chose the latter. The struggle wasn't worth the toll it took on him. He and Mom had never had an argument that involved any physical action more serious than a hairbrush flung at the refrigerator—I never did understand exactly why that took place, but I remember tension was high in the aftermath—and he was not ready now to try to control her unreasonable behavior with physical strength. If Mom was putting herself in any kind of physical danger, as on the night she decided to walk barefoot in the dark parking lot, he would restrain her. Otherwise, he would at last give up. Furious because she was ruining furniture, crushed by the ugliness of her words and the cold anger of her eyes, he'd just give up.

"All right," he would say, hands in the air as he backed away. "Go ahead. Sit wherever you want. Ruin anything you want. I don't care."

Individually and together, as the scene played itself out, Dad and I would try to change the expected outcome. We played good cop/bad cop. We talked about how much we were looking forward to having breakfast with her. Or we just prayed she would stop fighting us.

But midmornings often found Mom still sitting half-dressed, wet, and smelly on her couch in the den, staring silently at the wall opposite or speaking in loving tones to Charley-Dog about how mean Dad was, how ridiculous I was, how she was going to show "the big man" that she could do whatever she wanted to do and "Don't you worry, little Charley-Dog. Mama will take care of you."

As Dad sat silent at the table with his head in his hands, the television spewed noise and light that raced through the rooms of the house, crackling the tension that hung ready in the air. I would sit across the table from him, breathing fast, willing myself numb. With my gaze fastened on the mugs hanging on the wall behind my father's chair, I'd fall into prayer without even realizing it. When I became aware of the short desperate pleas threading through my mind, I'd stop, grasp the knots of faith hunkered down in my spirit, and start to pray again, consciously.

Eventually, convinced that time was the only help we could give Mom as she sat in her dark moods, Dad and I would look at each other.

"The sofa's been wet before, Daddy," I'd say. "We'll clean it up."

Then, more quietly, I'd remind him, "You know she always comes around. She'll be clean and dry in an hour or two or three...we'll just wait for the right time."

"Oh, I know, honey." His tone, too, was quiet. Though the television was loud and Charley was getting a talking-to from Mom about manners and being nice, she sometimes got upset that our conversation didn't include her.

So Dad continued in low tones spoken quickly from between his hunched shoulders. "And you know..." he'd go on.

Here it comes, I'd think. Hope. Hope was on its way, like a bright balloon, small but getting bigger.

"And you know," he'd say, "the days aren't all this way. This doesn't happen very often." His voice would get a little lighter. "And the whole day's not lost. In fact, by this afternoon she might be saying 'I love you, Daddy. I just don't know what I'd do without you.' We'll just wait a while. Maybe I can get her to drink some juice."

And there it was. Once again. The miracle of hope. The drive to try again. By the kindness of heaven and the power of the Almighty, my father never lost it. He conceded a battle sometimes, but he always returned to the field. He remained a valiant, loving, fierce warrior throughout Mom's illness. He fought for her. He fought to keep her alive, to keep her at home, to keep her with him. Hope helped him fight. He never let it go.

So we'd wait for the right time. Playing things low-key and casual was the safest and most reliable way to earn Mom's cooperation. If she didn't respond well at the beginning of a situation, we didn't press her any further. We would wait, forcing ourselves to be patient, taking care of each other as we worried and wondered. What if bedtime came and she was still sitting there? What could we try this time?

"How about some juice?"

"Some tea, Mama?"

"Come look at this squirrel out the window!"

Any one of these verbal weather balloons launched in her direction at the right moment could turn the forecast from stormy to stable. At worst she would ignore us.

But the easy comments or questions sent out every few minutes seemed to help. I imagined Mom caught up in clouds of confusion, swept away by anger, and left in an uncomfortable position from which she could find no escape. Maybe our words gave her the chance to start over.

In reality, I'm sure the working of her mind, moods, and emotions followed no such predictable path. For years Dad and I searched for some kind of pattern, some trace of cause and effect in Mom's behavior. We found very little. The most we could determine was the benefit of keeping her alert and as involved as possible in activity or conversation. The foggier her mind was— and a night's sleep left it foggy indeed—the worse her mood was.

Perhaps as she sat alone with her anger on those difficult mornings, she simply woke up a bit more. Maybe she just forgot all about how she ended up sitting alone on a damp cushion in the living room. Maybe it was simply Dad's loving and stubborn hope being blessed and rewarded once again. Maybe it was my prayers being answered.

Because sooner or later, Mom would blink. Budge. Answer. Smile. Move. Something. Something that led us to try again. To start all over as though it were nine o'clock instead of eleven or noon or later. Another offer of something to eat or drink, undivided attention to discovering her needs and desires, perhaps even some girlie giggling over what to wear today.

"Where is your sweater, Mama? I know you want that."

"Oh, yes, child. My sweater."

Hope filled the day's balloon, and Dad and I would watch it float up. Holding on to each other and to the gossamer string of our hope, we would take Mom's hand and step out in faith, back into living, following the balloon.

NOTES

- Morning—getting out of bed, into the bathroom and into clean clothes—was usually the most difficult part of my mother's day. We could never predict how the day would begin. However, a difficult morning did not always signal that the whole day would be hard.

- Mornings are an excellent time to have help in caregiving. Assistance getting the day started would have made the whole day easier for my father and me.

- We found that a low-key, casual approach was most successful in winning Mom's cooperation. Usually, the more intense we became, the more agitated she grew. Although it wasn't always easy to control our anxieties, most often we found success when we approached a situation as though we had no doubt of a successful outcome.

- As mentioned in the first chapter, especially in the early stages of the disease, we found that keeping Mom involved in activity or conversation kept her mood more positive. Her mind seemed foggiest first thing in the morning, or when she dozed off and awoke in the middle of the day.

- In our experience, hope always won. Every day.

Everything Old Is New Again

Forget the former things; do not dwell in the past. See, I am doing a new thing! Now it springs up; do you not perceive it? I am making a way in the wilderness, and streams in the wasteland.

—ISAIAH 43:18–19, NIV

Mom watched Dad and me talking as though she were watching a tennis match. The court was the round table where the three of us spent so many hours of business or pleasure or, sometimes, periods of loud arguing and desperate, killing silences. But as medication began to ease Mom's depression, the stormy days were fewer. Conversation flowed more freely, more often, filling in the gaps between the news shows Dad sought unceasingly on television.

Mom was usually a spectator in the conversation matches. Almost always she was at least one volley behind, turning her head so slowly that she was often looking at Dad as I was speaking, and vice versa. At times, she fancied herself the referee, suddenly interrupting our talk with an opinion or observation clearly intended to decide the matter she had in mind. And sometimes, surprisingly, the matter in her mind was also the matter Dad and I were discussing. Though such lucid conversations were few, they were invariably…interesting.

"I need to order the seeds for my tomatoes," Dad said. The day was a messy landscape, painted with a palette of cold grays, the canvas refusing to dry under thick brushstrokes. "It's almost the end of January. Usually I have seeds by now. I need potting soil, too. Maybe I'll mix my own again this year." My father's winters were spent planning for his springs.

"What varieties are you thinking about?" I asked him. "Last year the Celebrities did great. I guess you'll plant them again? What else?"

I knew this question would prompt a full-scale review of the seed catalogs. Sure enough, Dad reached over to the rainbow stack of booklets resting within his arm's reach. The sheets of thin paper bound with staples displayed a cornucopia of vegetables growing profusely in perfectly planted gardens. Other pages were covered with an Eden of flowers, blooming shrubs, flowering trees.

Magnifying glass in hand, Dad bent his head to the catalog. His nose was even closer to the print than usual. The inevitable criticism was coming, I knew.

"Why do they make it so hard to see which ones are good for our part of the country? You know—you just know—there are some poor people out there who order one of these kinds that just shrivel up and die in our heat! It's a good thing I know my tomatoes! Okay, Katrinka. Will you make me a list of these numbers so we can fill out the order form?"

"I'm ready!" Pencil in hand, I glanced up at Mom. Stretching so far across the table her head almost touched Dad's, she was doing her best to see the booklet he was studying.

"No, hang on a minute, Daddy." I reached to the stack for another catalog and handed it to Mom. She sat back and grinned, but said nothing.

Like spring showers, Dad's pronouncements of varieties and numbers were intermittent. Each one seemed to startle Mom for a second. Her head bounced up and down from the bright pages of her book to her observation of our tomato conversation, then wagged back and forth from my father to me as we discussed the relative merits of heat-tolerant varieties.

Then, suddenly, "Peppers!" Mom's voice was the equivalent of a sudden crack of thunder.

"What?" Dad's head jerked up and his magnifying glass dropped to the table.

"Peppers!" she repeated. "Tomatoes and peppers. I want peppers. Green peppers."

"Well, by all means!" Dad almost giggled with delight. "Peppers! Of course! Thank you for reminding us!"

The pepper remark and others like it—easy, confident words that fit snugly and rationally into the talk of the day—were like bright yellow paint splashed against a gray landscape. They were a source of glee and encouragement for days following, a shot of adrenaline for Dad and me, repeated to each other and reported to the doctor, to family, to all who asked how Mom was doing.

Of course her ability to make such verbal connections gradually diminished. And in the cruel way of Alzheimer's, her desire to participate remained after the ability had gone. Still, on her best days, she was able to adapt. I marveled at the way her mind and the Lord's power worked together to help her stay present with us.

Mom's usual entrée to a conversation was to decide that something— and it might be anything—was new.

Sitting in her chair at the table in the late afternoon or early evening, she would watch Dad and me talking. The tentative smile of morning would slowly spread wide across her face. As she raised her eyebrows, it appeared to me she was searching for a way to join the conversation.

Finally, she'd break in with the very safest word she knew to say. "Daddy!" she would call to my father.

"Yes, baby!" he would boom, with an exaggerated enthusiasm that betrayed his wariness. Eager as we were to have Mom participate in life, we were never sure what would come next.

"I'm talking to you," she might say, turning to me now with the still broad smile.

No more words yet. We would wait. Finally, shifting her feet back and forth, she'd continue.

"I see your blouse. Is it new?"

Probably it was an old sweatshirt I'd worn because I planned to do some cleaning. Maybe it was stretched out and holey. But a good day was a good day, and on a good day, even a worn-out sweatshirt could be a pretty blouse. And not just that. Also a blessing. A miracle.

So I would smile at her and watch the sun suffuse her face as I answered. "Oh, thank you, Mama! I've had this for a long time. I just don't wear it very often."

"Oh," she would breathe and then, running short on words, she'd smile and smile and shuffle and shuffle until I rescued her by asking, "Do you like it?"

"Oh, yes, child." Armed now with more words, she would look across at Dad. "Do you like that blouse, Daddy?" Then, turning back to me, "Is it new?"

Since just about anything could be new to Mom on any given day, there were lots of "new" conversations.

As she became unsteady walking, my father put a rail on the back porch steps. Mom seldom failed to mention it as she went up or down. "Your father made this for me. It's new. He put it right into this stuff," and she would pat the brick.

The rose garden Dad and I planted was perennially new, not from season to season or week to week, but from day to day, hour to hour, whenever she chanced to recognize it.

For a while, even my husband's hair was new. It turned gray when he was only about forty. Mom always loved the silvery color. But when she'd been ill for a few years, one day his hair was brand new to her. She couldn't tell him often enough how much she liked it.

Again and again she said, "I like your hair, Harold. Is that a new color?"

And Harold grinned and said, "Yes, ma'am. Your daughter gave it to me." The joke evaded her grasp, of course, but Harold laughed and so she laughed and then we all laughed. A few minutes passed and then she was rocking a bit and looking for a way into the conversation again. Again she seized on Harold's hair.

We laughed every time. Perhaps some tiny but well-used connection remained in her brain for a while after so many other connections had snapped or had been smothered and died. Maybe that tiny connection told her that noticing something new and complimenting someone about it was a good thing to do and smiles resulted. Maybe she remembered.

Long after the diagnosis of Alzheimer's had been made, long after we had grown tired of the same old things being seen as new time and again, long after we had become intimately acquainted with the daily ironies of *using* the forgetting, Dad and I found *ourselves* struggling to remember. *Remember* that pouring orange juice into the plate of eggs was not recognized as making a mess. *Remember* that refusing to go to bed had more to do with fright than willfulness. *Remember* that when she told us wild stories of someone trying to break into the house, Mom felt she was speaking absolute truth, so her anger at being contradicted was justified. *Remember* that her remarking again and again on the "new" plastic flowers—dusty and stiff in the old, cracked vase on the bureau—was her way of continuing to relate to her world, striving to be a part of our lives, to see and say what mattered to her and hear, please God, that it mattered to us as well.·

As I tried to keep her mind active with sight and sound and conversation, I finally realized I should speak to Mom as she spoke to me. Not only using simple words and very short sentences, but even choosing the subjects she chose.

And so, as tired as we all had become of hearing the same "new" questions and giving the same "new" answers again and again, I began to *initiate* the "new" exchanges and let her respond. Sometimes she could answer, sometimes not, but those well-worn talks were the most comfortable for her, bringing a smile or at least keeping the panic out of her eyes.

"Oh, look, Mama! A surprise for us outside! Roses!"

"What a pretty tablecloth this is! Is it new?"

"Wow! Shamrocks on your shoes! I love them!"

When we spoke to her of "new" things in the old familiar ways, we were able to keep Mom away from that place of darkness and confusion that I saw looming in her eyes. It was only my own speculation, of course, but I thought I could tell when she was looking into that yawning pit. I could imagine the cold breath that swept up from it, powerful and terrifying. She would open her mouth and close it, move her feet back and forth and jerk her head and shoulders back, trying to say or do something. Trying, it seemed to me, to exercise some control, to make some impact on her surroundings, to feel strong, safe. If she was unsuccessful, she retreated, away from the confusion surrounding her. Away from us, the suddenly sinister strangers who appeared to be blocking her escape. I could never decide who was more vulnerable in those grim moments: Mom, who knew no whats or whys but only gazed down into the emptiness, or the rest of us who knew that Alzheimer's was the monster that lived down there, slowly pulling her into the nothingness.

Anything that saved Mom from that void was a blessing. Keeping her engaged in some pleasantness of the here and now was one fairly reliable rescue. And even if the pleasantness of the here and now had been discussed an hour ago and a day ago and many times before that, the miracle was that we could so often cheer her with it, even in the later years of her illness. We could remember what she had noticed and liked in the past and help her notice it again. We could trick the disease, make it work against itself. We could help my mother win.

NOTES

▸ I realized early on that my father and I tended to overlook Mom in conversations. Her difficulty in keeping up, in finding the right words or sometimes any words at all made that oversight seem natural. But I knew from experience that keeping Mom connected to the present moment diminished the cloud of confusion that could settle over her without warning. And keeping her active in normal home and family activities for as long as possible was enjoyable to all of us.

▸ Conversation is challenging and becomes more so as Alzheimer's progresses. Probably the simplest way to help your loved one stay engaged is to follow her lead. Be aware of what attracts her attention in a positive way; you could even make a list. Talk about those things. Give her time to respond, but even if she doesn't, keeping her attention focused on something pleasant will benefit everyone.

➤ Look at your loved one as you talk, even when she isn't part of the conversation. Simple eye contact seemed to be pleasant and reassuring to Mom.

➤ My father and I found great success by speaking to my mother as she spoke to us: in short sentences, slowly, using easy words. Sometimes asking simple questions worked; other times questions appeared to cause her anxiety. Trial and error was definitely the order of every day.

➤ Conversation with Mom was time-consuming. But even when time was short, I talked to her as I moved through the house doing other things. As long as it didn't anger her, I found that, even when she didn't participate, talking to her gave *me* pleasure.

The Kindness of Strangers

Then the righteous will answer him, "Lord, when did we see you...a stranger and invite you in, or needing clothes and clothe you? When did we see you sick or in prison and go to visit you?" The King will reply, "Truly I tell you, whatever you did for one of the least of these brothers and sisters of mine, you did for me."

—MATTHEW 25: 37–40, NIV

When my sister and I were little and Mom wasn't pleased with our choice of clothes, she used to tell us we looked like we'd been "called for and couldn't make it." I heard it more often than my sister, since I seemed to have significantly less talent for putting together an acceptable ensemble.

To me, in fact, Mom went beyond the called-for-and-couldn't-make-it assessment. "Child," she would say, shaking her head, "you look like the wreck of the Hesperus."

Presumably the Hesperus was a ship. That had a bad day at sea. And wrecked. Sank, or broke into pieces, or at the very least took on water. I picture a certain sogginess. Seaweed was probably involved.

That image, not just the wreck but the entire voyage of the Hesperus, sometimes flashed through my mind as my parents and I left the house to venture out in public. Being in public with Mom was an adventure. From beginning to end.

I drove my parents somewhere almost every day. Dad could drive short distances to places he was familiar with, but his bad eyesight

54

meant he needed a driver to get everywhere else. And since he wouldn't allow anyone to stay with Mom, she was always along for the ride. The itinerary was determined by my parents' needs—stamps, groceries, prescriptions, birdseed, or simply my father's need to get out of the house for a while.

The trip we made most often was to breakfast. During the mildest stage of her illness, Mom had grown accustomed to eating breakfast out. Sticking with familiar routines made life easier as the Alzheimer's progressed, so most mornings found the three of us preparing to go to the supercenter. My parents loved the place. Only five minutes from their house, the store not only could supply most of their needs, but also housed a little cafe in one corner. It served breakfast sandwiches in the morning and pizza 'til closing time. Mom wanted to eat there every day.

Getting her dressed was the first challenge. Even early on, Mom's choice of clothing was questionable, so going out required some extra preparation.

Shoes, for example. Barefoot was okay at home, but the supercenter frowned on customers with bare feet.

Dad would start the reminders at least half an hour before we were to leave the house. "Shoes, honey! Here are your sunglasses! Would you like me to carry them? No? In your pocket? Will they fit in there with all those tissues? Okay! Okay fine! But you don't even have your sweater on yet. Okay! Okay fine." Five minutes later, "Shoes, honey!" again. Either Dad or I had to help her put them on. So I guess the reminders were for me.

"What did you say, Daddy?" Mom would ask. The look on her face was as blank as her feet were bare. The rest of the conversation wasn't likely to add anything in either case.

"Your shoes, honey! Your shoes! Time to get them on! Let's go get some breakfast!"

"Where are my shoes, Daddy?"

"Right there by your feet! I brought them to you thirty minutes ago!"

About this time, Mom would be moving last night's dinner napkin to various spots on the table, looking under it for the thing—she knew not what—my father wanted her to find. Before he noticed and reacted to the napkin navigation, I usually managed to step in, finding her shoes as if by magic.

"Oh, look, Mama! Here they are! Your good ol' tennis shoes! Let me help you. We'll be really fast doing it together!"

If it was a good day, she would grin and stick a foot in my face and we'd laugh. If not, putting on her shoes could take a while.

"O-*kay!* Great!" Dad rejoiced at the completion of each step of the long departure process. "You got your shoes on! Now— where is your sweater?"

Winter and summer, Mom wore that green sweater. If she wouldn't let me help her put it on, it hung twisted across her shoulders, caught up in folds that made it too short but sometimes served to hide the hole from a cigarette burn that had somehow made it to the sweater's back. The pockets were stuffed with tissues and paper napkins that she squirreled away, fanatically, ferociously, at every opportunity. In the seam of one shoulder was a hole I mended repeatedly, always after she went to bed. A month or so later, the hole would reappear, letting the color of her blouse show through like a patch on a clown's costume or an angel sitting on her shoulder.

Still, raggedy as it was, that sweater was usually the most chic component of Mom's attire. To win a smile from her, I often told her how lovely it was. What she wore *under* the sweater called to mind the wreck of the Hesperus. My mother, the beauty of so many photographs, could no longer dress herself. Though she made it clear she didn't appreciate our assistance, most days she would eventually succumb to our efforts to help her. Still, she insisted on wearing only certain shirts, most with holes burned in them from the cigarettes she refused to give up. Loose-fitting pants were a necessity because they were easier to get on and off and up and down, and didn't show the bulky outline of disposable underwear. The pants, too, were often scorched by a dropped cigarette. So this woman who had loved clothes and shoes and matching handbags for the first sixty years of her life, who had walked with grace and exhibited the formal manners of her English mother, came at last to be quite another sight when she went to town. The Hesperus itself could scarcely have been more eye-catching. As we strove to get through each morning, walking the perilously thin and sharp edge of her moods, we were pleased simply to have her warm, dry, and modest when we left the house.

At last, another "O-*kay!*" from Dad. His bellow held equal parts relief and enthusiasm to have the day off to a start at last. "Let's go see Mike and Shaun!"

With me in the driver's seat, Dad riding co-pilot, and Mom in the back asking for cigarettes or fiddling endlessly with the seatbelt she never allowed us to fasten, we set out for the supercenter. The little café in the corner was a miraculous affair in its own right. It was actually a pizza shop, owned and run by a husband and wife from Pakistan whose names sounded neither Pakistani nor Italian. For five or six years before I met them, I heard my parents speak of Mike and Shaun, always in the tone one reserves for good friends, which was surprising since my parents had few friends. Six days a week, Mike and Shaun served breakfast sandwiches and coffee early in the morning before the pizza rush began. My parents were regulars. As I joined the breakfast ritual, I soon shared my parents' fondness and respect for Mike and Shaun.

From my father's favorite parking spot in the handicapped section, it was a short walk to the side entrance of the store. Dad strode ahead. Mom and I walked far behind, often with her arm wound across mine. Her hair was matted to her head, brushed but not clean. Her dentures, too, were dirty. Mom's jaws were incredibly strong when she decided she didn't want a toothbrush in her mouth, and the challenge of getting the dentures out and then back in was so difficult that I attempted it rarely, only on the most congenial of days.

I wondered what people in the store thought of me when they saw Mom's clothes and hair and, on her happy mornings, the toothy grin she bestowed on one and all. During the early days of watching her shuffle along in holey clothes and those white tennis shoes dotted with green shamrocks, I had to struggle to keep from crying. The tears sprang partly from vivid childhood memories of hearing her admonish me about my own appearance—"Stand up straight, child, and be proud!"— and partly, I admit, from embarrassment. The embarrassment wore off.

The greeter at the door spoke brightly to Mom, as one would speak to a child. I was surprised to find that employees throughout the store recognized my parents. Most of them seemed to know intuitively when and how to speak to my mother.

By the time we reached the café counter, Dad was already pouring coffee from a coffee maker that sat within his reach. There was no need to order; Mike and Shaun were already preparing "the usual." One or both of them would be talking to my father, about the weather or sports or their sons or his grandchildren, but when Mom appeared, their focus shifted immediately to her.

"Good morning, young lady!" Mike exclaimed, his smile revealing his own bad teeth and a heart the size of Texas. "You're so beautiful today!"

Sometimes, "Thank you!" was Mom's reply; sometimes, "Oh! You, too!" And sometimes she just shuffled past, with or without a smile.

After he brought us our coffees, Dad returned to the counter for more conversation while he waited for the sandwiches. Mom and I always sat at the same table, midway down the side wall—except on those highly irritating and therefore tense occasions when other customers had chosen to sit there.

I was continually amazed at how easily Mom expressed herself when she was angry. In a loud voice, she'd start a litany of critical comments: "What are they doing there? Look how slow they're eating. That man looks silly. He should take his hat off. What on earth is she wearing? That child's hands are filthy." Fortunately, her comments seemed to take all her strength, so she didn't fight my hand on her elbow as I guided her to another table, as far away as possible from other diners.

The wait for the food was never long. Mom spent the time looking around and folding napkins to put in her pockets, while I sat and thought about how familiar and even comforting the scent of this place had become. The strange aroma, blended of pizza spices, bacon, coffee, and bleach-laced cleaning solution, could usually overcome whatever less-pleasant smells might cling to my mother's clothes and person.

The breakfast sandwiches—eggs with cheese and ham layered on buttery soft croissants—were served on thin paper plates. Somehow Dad managed to carry all three at once without dropping anything. Mom's plate always came with a knife and fork. Dad had requested them only once, he told me; thereafter, Mike and Shaun remembered. Even from behind the counter, they could probably see how difficult it was for Mom to chew. Her dentures no longer fit, but she refused to go to a dentist, and since she maintained a healthy weight, we saved our strength for more critical battles. Still, eating was a slow and sometimes, I feared, painful process for her. So Mike and Shaun always sent a knife and fork, along with some extra napkins. Mom folded the napkins while my engineer father cut her sandwich into uniformly-sized bites.

Many days, Shaun—beautiful, quiet, graceful, with warm dark eyes—came to the table and put her hand on Dad's shoulder, then looked across at Mom. In her musical accent she would ask, "How are you, Mama?" She seldom got a response, but she always waited, just in case. On her conversational days, Mom would hold up one finger while she chewed. And chewed. And chewed. When Dad wriggled in discomfort at the long delay, Shaun would pat his shoulder and continue to look expectantly at my mother, who would, finally, swallow. Looking at Shaun with a slow smile, she would breathe a single word, "Fine," and take another bite.

Eating seemed to take even longer at the café than at home. We tried to be patient. We knew that to hurry Mom was to risk not only her anger, but also what might be her only full meal for the day. So we waited while she talked about all those things over there with pictures on them—"Those are cans, Mama. Full of popcorn! Aren't they pretty?"—and while she pointed wordlessly to the baby sitting in a highchair at a table across the room, and while she interrupted her chewing to fold one more napkin— "Oh, by all means, yes! Put that in your pocket! You don't want to run out of napkins!"—this last uttered by Dad in a tone of frustrated sarcasm completely lost on Mom. Finally she would finish each and every carefully sliced bite. Or simply stop eating and push the plate away.

Then it was time for the shopping. On the days when Mom declared she was too tired to walk, or just shook her head and folded her arms and refused to stand, Mike and Shaun were quick to suggest that she stay where she was. They would watch her from their counter while Dad and I split up to get the shopping done quickly.

But most days, especially early on, Mom came with us. She pushed the shopping cart as she always had, but now it supported her and helped her balance, much as a walker would. While Dad struck out on his own, chatting with employees here and there, Mom and I made our way slowly through the store. She'd swipe a grape or two in the produce department, sniff the artificial flowers with an appreciative smile, and lovingly stroke the stuffed animals in the toy department.

She liked to speak to strangers, telling a young mother, "Your little girl is such a good baby!" and suggesting to a man who looked to be in a hurry, "You need to smell those flowers! See? Right over there!"

I came to dread those encounters. The right words came to Mom more and more slowly. As I imagined the person she addressed was trying to escape or ignore her, I smiled hard with my mouth and pleaded for patience with my eyes. I filled in words as quickly and quietly as possible and sometimes even tugged gently on Mom's arm, trying to move her on. All the while I watched for signs that any part of the situation—the stranger, the words I chose, my effort to keep her moving—was becoming a source of irritation for her. Her anger could erupt in a second. I dreaded it at home; in public I *feared* it.

"What do you think you're talking about? Why are you here?" she might suddenly sneer, or sometimes she just began calling, "Daddy! Daddy! LJ! Come here, LJ! Hurry!"

Sometimes she simply jerked the cart with amazing strength, letting the clattering metal and tumbling contents express her anger. As difficult as such outbursts were at home, in public they felt like the beginning of the end of the world. The panic they provoked nauseated me.

The miracle, however, was that the panic passed quickly. A strength that I knew came from heaven revived me like oxygen. As far as I know, I was the only one who ever doubted I had the situation under control. I reacted in the same way I had managed emergencies and near disasters while raising three sons: with authority and calm.

Most of the time during these outbursts, I was able to simply get Mom moving again. The energy she expended in yelling or jerking the cart was generally all she could muster; her body followed me instinctively as I led her away. On the other side of grace, the stranger involved would move away also. To my knowledge, the other person never complained, not to me, not to anyone in the store. People seemed to understand, even in the space of a minute or two, that Mom had little control over her emotions and that moving out of her sight was the best remedy for the uproar.

In the months to come, I would find that, somehow, this was *always* the case. When we were out with Mom, children might stare, adults might give her a wide berth, but invariably, the strangers who came into closest contact with her were helpful and considerate. Either in their actions or their forbearance, through their words or their silence, they were kind.

The daily routine of a ride in the car, breakfast at the café in Mike and Shaun's corner, and a walk through the store became a source of comfort for Mom. Nothing else in her daily activities was as predictable as her satisfaction with breakfast at the supercenter. The time was good for Dad also. Some of the employees at the store became friends to him, people who sincerely cared about how he was feeling and what he was doing. They spoke to him when he most needed a moment or two of lucid conversation, and never, as far as I knew, made any reference to Mom's appearance or her erratic behavior.

Still, the anxiety remained with me whenever we were in public with Mom, a combination of fierce protectiveness and heavy dread, a remembrance of the self-possessed mother who raised me mixed with an acute awareness of the bent, dirty little woman walking at my side. With effort born of love, I reminded myself she was still my mother. And still the beauty my father adored.

Together, Dad and I walked through Alzheimer's with our guard up, watching for anything that could cause a problem for my mother. But gradually we learned to walk also with the expectation of strength and grace sufficient for the moment.

NOTES

> A sense of humor is vital in a home where Alzheimer's lives. Being able to see the comedy in, for instance, the series of non sequiturs that made up my parents' conversations was a lifeline for me. Sometimes we laughed at things that weren't so obviously funny, like the day Mom put her dentures in upside down, or the time she sneaked out of the house to go downtown and arrived back home in a tow truck. Disasters avoided were cause for laughter. Absurd situations were funny. Laughter dissolved some of the tension in the house; it was good for my spirit, Dad's, Mom's. It revived heavy hearts. It was a blessing for us all, a miracle that, as time passed, became more and more treasured.

> Sticking to familiar things and familiar routines was always easier than introducing something new to Mom. New places, new clothes, different foods, even a new medication—sure to be a different color or size or shape—Mom noticed all those things. And disliked them. Often vehemently. Even after the usual ways of doing things had clearly slipped from her conscious memory, the scenes, smells, and sounds of the supercenter didn't appear to cause her the same anxiety she exhibited when we took her somewhere she'd never been. Obviously, it's not possible to eliminate all new objects and experiences from your loved one's life, but when you have a choice, I'd try the familiar first.

> As Alzheimer's robbed Mom of her memory, I saw it also taking her judgment and inhibitions. She might say, do, or wear almost anything. Being aware of that reality didn't mean I was always ready to handle it, but it helped.

> "Clean, dry, and modest" is, in my experience, a worthy fashion goal for an Alzheimer's patient. Some loved ones may easily accept the processes and assistance necessary to go beyond that goal. But for patients like my mother and caregivers like me, trying to achieve more than clean, dry, and modest may not be worth the price likely to be paid in extreme effort and frustration.

➤ Caregivers would benefit from learning to *accept* help early on. You may find it difficult to say "yes" to assistance from the people you encounter by chance in a public place. For example, Dad accepted Mike and Shaun's help, but answered "Oh, we're fine" to strangers who offered to carry groceries or pointed out a place where Mom could sit and rest. Eventually, he needed help so often, he overcame his embarrassment, swallowed his pride and accepted such offers gratefully.

➤ I was always successful in managing Mom's public outbursts. But I didn't do it with words; words rarely calmed her down. Instead, the best strategy was to move her away from the situation. Sometimes that was easy; sometimes, difficult. It was never impossible. One tactic that worked for me was to put one hand on Mom's elbow and the other on the opposite shoulder, guiding her firmly away from the situation, with no thought for apology and no concern for shopping yet to be done. Knowing in advance what you will do is a source of strength. Having a plan allows you to do what is necessary without distraction or fear.

➤ But also be aware that having a plan doesn't make it okay to throw caution to the wind. For example, a caregiver shouldn't expect always to be able to control a loved one who is bigger, heavier, or stronger. If Mom had been bigger than I, I wouldn't have taken her to an unfamiliar place on my own unless it was an emergency. Common sense should tell us not to put ourselves or our loved ones in a questionable situation, no matter how much success we've had in the past.

➤ In caring for someone with Alzheimer's, I believe caregivers must choose their battles. Some patients are endlessly cooperative, but others, like my mother, fight many things. Doctor's visits, for example, or maybe any visit. For those patients, caregivers must determine the relative importance of activities. What is necessary? What is desirable? What seemed like a good idea, but is really unnecessary?

- > Be alert to ways your loved one can exercise safely. Mom didn't want to walk and she refused to use a walker, but she would walk through the store, pushing a grocery cart that served well as a walker.

- > Embarrassment at the appearance or actions of a loved one with Alzheimer's is understandable. It doesn't label a caregiver as hardhearted or disrespectful. But embarrassment *is* an unnecessary burden to carry. Alzheimer's and other forms of dementia are so common today that most people are not surprised by their physical effects. In my experience with Mom, people were never hurtful in word or action. They were understanding, even kind. Coming to that expectation sooner rather than later will be a great advantage to you and to your loved one.

The Rose Garden

The Lord is my shepherd, I lack nothing. He makes me lie down in green pastures, he leads me beside quiet waters, he refreshes my soul.
—PSALM 23:1–3, NIV

At the height of Mom's illness, my father and I planted a rose garden.

Dad had spoken of roses many times since the big old hickory tree died, quickly, from no visible disease, no identifiable cause. Just one day the trunk snapped a few feet from the ground, revealing its hollow core.

Together Dad and I wondered if we had missed something— were there fewer leaves than the year before? Were they paler? Misshapen? We couldn't remember, hadn't even noticed, until the day the tree fell and left a hole in the lawn where we dug up the stump.

It was, at least, a sun-filled hole. Still, my father mourned the loss of the tree, inspected its neighbors carefully, worried about them.

Every time someone mentioned replacing the tree, he was noncommittal.

"Welllll…." He stretched the word, making it climb to the high tones of indecision instead of letting it fall to finality. Sometimes he added, "That would be a good place for a rose garden." Once or twice he used different words, like "I always wanted a rose garden in this lawn." But that was all—only words. To me, his tone said the time to plant roses had long since passed.

Dad and I often walked over the lawn, identifying limbs to be pruned from the crepe myrtles, searching out crabgrass to be sprayed. Mom never wanted to join us, but as we went from shrubs to flowerbeds to a weedy patch of grass, I kept my eyes moving, looking right, left, behind us, like a driver in heavy traffic, watching for her. Just in case she changed her mind.

If she decided she needed us, her usual practice was to stand just inside the doorway and shout.

"Daddy! Daddy! Daddy!"

He would go to her and stand with her at the screen door. He wore a soft hat on his bald head to protect him from the sun and his "mudders" on his feet, so he was prepared for any task the lawn might thrust upon him. But it was difficult to be prepared for Mom's needs. They were as unpredictable as the Texas weather and could change with lightning speed.

So Dad could only listen. With her inside and him outside, he listened through the screen door as her fear shaped stories about a man who tried to steal the car or a bill that was so long overdue, she and Dad would soon be homeless. Of course there was no man; the bills were paid; but in Mom's mind these catastrophes were living among us like monsters.

My father listened, or if Mom called me, I listened, and one of us would propose solutions for the current dilemma. One after another we'd pitch them out there, until sometimes, having heard some magic word of comfort, Mom's face would soften, brighten. With a smile, she might say, "Oh, that's right! So it's just fine, isn't it? Oh! Thank you so much!" And we'd walk her to her favorite spot on the green velvet sofa to doze until the monsters came again.

But too often Mom heard no magic in our words. Her growing frustration set her eyes on fire and made her feet move as if the floor were burning. Finally her words would explode. "Just forget it! Forget it! I don't care anyway. I'm tired. Forget it!"

Sometimes the monster was some imagined hurt we had inflicted on her. At those times she fought us right there on the front porch—Dad, me, or both of us. First with words spit through clenched jaws, then, on the darkest days, with fists flying into the screen and feet kicking at the door. We defended ourselves with the only weapons we could conjure up: shocked faces, desperate denials, exhausted apologies. At last, when we had nothing else to offer her, we gave our despair, me with tears, my father with pleading. But she'd hurl her own despair back at us, and hers always won. Defeated, we'd watch as she stomped barefoot across the floor and fell onto the sofa, making no effort to catch her body, her arms slack, her usually pale face still flushed with anger.

Even with such formidable challenges, I don't know why I didn't propose it sooner. "Let's just make a rose garden, Daddy."

When I finally did introduce the idea, I heard myself using the tactic I regularly employed to gain Mom's cooperation: the strategy of multiple persuasions.

"Let's just make a rose garden, Daddy. Why not? Why shouldn't we? Let's do it! It'll be great! Where do we start?"

I felt my face smiling. I heard my voice smiling. The questions fairly bounced out of my mouth. The miracle was that Dad listened. Instead of dodging the bright balls of my enthusiasm, he caught them.

Then he laughed out loud and, slapping his thigh, said, "O-*kay*, Katrinka! Let's do it!"

Mom reacted with her usual enthusiasm. "Oh, here, here! Cut that out! That's just too much!"

Maybe I hadn't made this suggestion earlier because somewhere down in my subconscious I knew what this rose garden would require. The right soil, plants suited to Texas, a little spray for black spot—roses! Right? Oh, my heavens no!

For my father, nothing was simple. A simple row of radish seeds required a spading fork, a rake, a hoe, two posts, string, a yardstick and tape measure, and a week's worth of research into the best variety of seed for these red-bottomed, white-topped, keep-them-moist-or-they'll-be-tough-and-bitter little vegetables.

And this was not a radish garden we were planting. These were *roses*.

With Mom dozing and watching *Gunsmoke* on the couch, we began. First, the location: Dad surveyed the empty spot in the lawn from every angle to determine the sunniest placement.

Next, "A perfect square," Dad decided. No surprise there. Perfection was his goal in any project—indeed, in his life. A square, straight lines of equal length forming four equal angles, was a relatively straightforward way of achieving it, at least as far as shape was concerned.

With his trusty hoe extended at arm's length, Dad pointed. "Maybe just a little west of the hickory tree hole."

Construction of the planting area took us longer than we had anticipated. I could blame part of the delay on Dad's bad eyesight and his intolerance for any deviation from his original plan. But these elements were surely offset by his expertise in planning and his facility with tools of every description. So I'm forced to attribute some of the delays to his helper.

That would be…me.

"Get me that drill motor, will you, Katrinka?" he'd ask me.

Huh? Drill motor? The one attached to his drill? Did it come off? Wonder what you do with a drill motor other than use it on the drill?

"Here's your drill, Daddy," I replied. "I can't see how to get the motor off."

"What?!" My father's eighty-plus years' worth of impatience-tamed sometimes escaped through the force and decibels he could inject into a single word. So. I learned it was simply a matter of semantics. His "drill motor" was the *drill*.

And there was yet another cause for construction delays: many trips to the door to fight the monsters that plagued Mom. Some days the project stopped entirely, the trips to the door too numerous, the monsters too fierce. Or maybe Mom just wanted us inside instead of out.

Sometimes it did indeed seem too late to plant roses. The oft-repeated scenario of pulling out the tools, planning the amount of work we could reasonably expect to accomplish in a couple of hours, and then having the monsters steal even that small portion of the day—the frustration threatened to overwhelm us. In huge, loud, tearing bites or in tireless nipping and nibbling, Alzheimer's ate its way into our hope. We fought the fiends that lived in Mom's mind. We fought despair, hers and ours. We fought to keep her with us and sometimes we fought to escape her.

As late summer became fall, we worked when we could, digging up grass, turning over the soil, adding more to elevate the close-to-perfect square of black earth a few inches above the surrounding ground. Falling leaves gradually covered the lawn. Though the grass remained green beneath the multi-hued blanket, cooler temperatures stopped its growth. Caught between summer and winter, the grass hung on. Not growing, but not giving up. Not yet.

Surprises popped up as the project progressed. One afternoon I found Dad standing over a pile of railroad ties at the back of the storage shed. My parents had scavenged them from a section of abandoned train track twenty years earlier. Now Dad gazed down at them as if they were a priceless treasure.

"Look at these, Katrinka! They'll hold that new soil in place. A perfect border!"

The ties did indeed look just right. They also looked heavier than lead. Dad, however, said weight wasn't a problem. He and Mom had moved the timbers twenty years ago; surely he and I could do it now. Alas! He was mistaken. The twenty years hadn't added weight to the wood, Dad said, so apparently I wasn't as strong as Mom had been. Yes, yes, I agreed. That explained the problem. But...what to do?

When strength failed, science saved us. Happy as a clam, Dad applied the laws of physics to the problem, then devised tools to help us roll, pull, and lever the timbers into position. I applied encouragement, determination, and my dread of disappointing him.

Eventually, the ties were laid, angles squared, and soil leveled. Dad's expectations for the project were met, so far; the bed was a masterpiece, with dark soil made especially for roses rising above the lawn where the hickory tree used to be. At last it was time to select and plant the roses. Most would be red, because, according to my father, "roses should just be red." Besides, red was Mom's favorite color. We also purchased a couple of yellow ones, out of deference to me—and Texas.

The plants struggled a bit at first. One died. The variety named "Mr. Lincoln" turned out to be an impostor we dubbed "John Wilkes Booth."

But they bloomed. And, chosen for their fragrance as well as for their color and hardiness, the flowers scented the lawn like a breeze from heaven.

Every time she came outside, we called them to Mom's attention. Some days she refused to look in their direction. With a growl, she'd declare, "I don't see any flowers."

But on other days, the roses delighted her. Each time she took notice of them, they were new to her. Again and again. Each time, she was astonished to hear they did indeed belong to us.

"How lovely!" she would say, or "Isn't that nice?" A minute or two after Dad had shown them to her, she'd turn back to him. "Daddy!" she'd say in a shocked tone. "Did you see these flowers?"

Black spot and mildew came and went. We sprayed, fed, watered, and sprayed again. Sometimes insects ate into the buds, but even then, the fragrance remained.

Dad tended those roses like children, determined they should be perfect. Showpieces. And he was pleased with them, I'm sure. But as I look back, I don't think they ever quite measured up to the full extent of his hopes. Too tall, not bushy enough, curled leaves here, a scorched one there. So he worked on them, determined to cure their ills and give them the best possible place to thrive. I'm sure it was the work that pleased him. The taking care.

For me, the blossoms were enough. The beauty of the flowers made even the thorns acceptable. With regal grace, tall on their stems, they tolerated storm and sun, insect and disease, relying on their irresistible and unquenchable fragrance when their appearance was less than perfect.

And more often than we had any right to expect, there would come a perfect blossom, lovely as a smile. Petal by petal it would open. Unaware of our admiration it would reign, until time passed and, petal by petal, the blossom fell from air to earth.

But even when all the petals had dropped and the flower's stem stood bare, I wouldn't let go. Surely something so grand could not simply *not be.* Surely some still-fragrant vestige could be saved a while longer. So I scooped up the fallen petals and put them in a clear glass bowl. Their scent remained for a long time, a faint reminder of the beauty the blooms had lavished on us.

The rose garden was a good project. For Dad, something to plan for and take care of. For Mom, a surprise without mystery or threat. And for me, beauty to be held and inhaled and saved. Those roses.

NOTES

> Be aware of your own health—mental and physical. Obviously, not everyone will react to the demands of caregiving in the same way, but be aware that stress and long hours take a toll on the body and the mind. I paid attention when Dad started losing weight, and his reluctance to plan and engage in new activities was a big red flag. I talked to him about his feelings and asked him to consider whether he might be depressed. He consulted his doctor; together they worked on a treatment plan. As you monitor your loved one's health, be sure to watch your own as well.

> Dad had always loved to dig into handyman projects. But time spent exclusively with Alzheimer's seemed to dry up his creativity and smother his initiative. When I saw his life shrinking to match the dimensions of Mom's, I knew I had to search for ways he could get away. Dad's poor eyesight complicated the situation, but one of the easiest and most pleasant activities for him was going to lunch with his brother once a week. To discover your own options, brainstorm with friends, other Alzheimer's caregivers, the staff and volunteers at your senior center or at your church.

> "Getting away" need not mean leaving your loved one, although it might consist of that. But getting away can mean many things that require, at most, someone to come in who will simply alert you if your loved one has a critical need. Cell phones and neighbors are a powerful combination—they can give you an hour at the library, an afternoon with a friend, a walk around the block, a movie.

➤ Getting away can also mean just doing what you want to do while your loved one looks on. For a while, I felt guilty when I pulled out my crocheting instead of doing something useful, like rubbing lotion on Mom's hands. But when I felt myself relaxing, when I felt my spirits rise, I realized that taking care of myself made me *more* able to improve Mom's quality of life.

Lean on Me

Each one will be like a shelter from the wind and a refuge from the storm, like streams of water in the desert and the shadow of a great rock in a thirsty land. Then the eyes of those who see will no longer be closed, and the ears of those who hear will listen. The fearful heart will know and understand....
—ISAIAH 32:2–4, NIV

Before our trip to Colorado, I never imagined Dad would hide from anything out of fear. But of course, we're all afraid. Of something. Sometime.

After a few weeks of helping him care for Mom, I saw the fear Dad lived with. Surely afraid of the way his life might change if he acknowledged the dementia, he denied it for as long as possible. He hid Mom's bizarre behavior, black moods, and unreasonable demands from me and my sister for at least a couple of years. The tellers at the bank and the checkers at the grocery store—all those people who could see my parents in the unguarded moments— must have known Mom was ill long before I did.

But even as I saw that denying reality made life so much more difficult than it had to be for Dad, I found myself hiding, too. Dad never knew about the job offers I turned down in order to be there for him and Mom. I didn't tell him how disruptive the situation was to my family. And for long months after acknowledging the truth of the Alzheimer's diagnosis, I refused to admit a blinding truth: Dad and I needed help.

I bemoaned my situation to family and a few close friends, but for so long I could not see—or was reluctant to accept—that I had *chosen* my place smack in the middle of my parents' difficulties. They never asked me to step into their day-to-day lives. I alone had made Mom's illness my problem. And now *I* needed help to handle the gigantic challenges Alzheimer's poses, not just to its victims, but also to their families. I didn't see it at the time, but I was as stubborn as my father in resisting when my husband urged me to look for that help, look for any resources available to families living with Alzheimer's.

It took me months, for example, to force myself to attend an Alzheimer's support group meeting. The thought of sitting in a roomful of people just like me who were dealing with loved ones just like my mother literally nauseated me.

I had done it once. Soon after Mom's diagnosis, I went to a day-long seminar for personal and professional caregivers. I had to fight myself to go and then fought to make myself stay.

A large church in Dallas hosted the seminar. The trees that shaded areas of the asphalt parking lot were themselves succumbing to the heat of the summer day, pale leaves curling around their stems and branches hanging listless in the thick air. As I entered the meeting room, someone was closing the drapes on the hot light pouring in through walls of windows. The center of the large room was lined in chairs, rows of folding chairs, at least two hundred by my count. A fence of tables filled with notebooks, pamphlets, brochures, and books corralled the chairs on three sides. Standing at the tables, vendors smiled too brightly at the few brave souls who perused their materials. The professionals with name tags hanging from bright blue cords smiled and conversed at the front of the room. But most of the attendees, identified by the adhesive name tags stuck to our chests, looked shell-shocked.

The seminar provided a wealth of information about many aspects of caregiving: activities to stimulate thought and memory, the value of routines and schedules, exercises to help maintain coordination and muscle tone, the importance of diet and nutrition, information on critical legal and financial issues. The well-trained speakers were knowledgeable, experienced, prepared with handouts, and able to answer questions. The knowledge I gained in those hours might have been of immediate value to me—except that it scared me so badly I wanted to run away and forget all I had heard. I wanted to hide.

With a smile only face-deep, I shook hands with other attendees. But none of us really talked to each other. The speakers didn't invite any sharing of experiences and made no mention at all of the *emotional* toll of Alzheimer's on the patient's family and friends. No one spoke of what those of us out in the folding chairs might be *feeling*; no one said anything about shock, panic, or fear. No one mentioned confusion, except as it pertained to the Alzheimer's patients. And no one spoke of hope, humor, sweet moments, and good days. The emphasis was on practicality, coping, surviving. Entirely appropriate, but not encouraging.

At the end of the day, as I peeled off my name tag and walked out the door, I felt worse, not better. The people who had stood onstage and dispensed their information could take off their name tags and go home. But for the rest of us, Alzheimer's wouldn't peel off. I realize now that I wasn't able to take advantage of the wealth of resources offered that day because the diagnosis was still so fresh; I was still angry and afraid. I knew only that the seminar was not an experience I would choose again.

As months passed and Mom's condition continued to deteriorate, I sank deeper into the hole of isolation Dad had begun, years ago, to dig. Thinking it must offer him some kind of protection, I enlarged it to accommodate my fears also. Even when I recognized it as a cave I could easily get lost in, I refused to come out.

Meanwhile, my husband continued to gather information for me about Alzheimer's support groups. By this time, I had accepted a part-time job, a fifteen-hours-a-week oasis of order and predictability in my life. Even so, I could easily have managed to attend the meetings, which were held in several locations convenient to my home or my parents' home. But month after month, I refused to go. My husband must have despaired as he heard me parrot my father:

"We're doing okay."

"I just don't want to go."

"Things are manageable for now."

"I don't see how complaining to a bunch of other people can help—and I don't want to listen to them complain either."

When I finally did attend a meeting, it was the Five Minute Rule that got me there. The Five Minute Rule states that you can do anything for five minutes. You can try out some potentially distasteful activity for just five minutes, and if you're doing okay with it, you can stay for another five minutes. If not, you can leave.

My friend Judy, who introduced me to the Five Minute Rule, had been incredibly patient in bringing up the idea of attending the support group meetings. I was certain she, like my husband, could not possibly understand how wrong she was when she said sharing with others would be helpful.

"I'll go next month," was my standard reply.

But my friend was unbelievably persistent. She brought up the meetings so often, I finally began to weaken. The bright light that eventually melted my resistance was the shocking postscript she tacked on to each plea: "Please just give it a try. I'll go with you."

Maybe I went to get her and my husband off my back about it. Maybe I went because I wanted her to see what I thought I already knew: the meetings would be mostly gripe sessions. Whatever the reason, I went. For five minutes.

The early fall sky was still bright when I arrived a half hour ahead of time. Lingering Texas heat filled the car as I sat in the parking lot looking at the church building where the group met. I had already driven around it once, trying to decide which door to enter. When another car parked and a couple of ladies walked in, I followed. I followed them right up to the door of the church's gymnasium where they were going to work out. Wondering if my five minutes were over yet, I asked the man at the gym's scheduling desk about the Alzheimer's support group meeting. He directed me to the library, around the corner at the end of the hall.

A small group gathered slowly. Eventually, six of us sat on a couch and chairs beside long rows of metal bookshelves. The scent of books filled the air; usually a comforting smell, on this night, it left me cold.

The room was beige: the walls were beige, the tables were beige, the couch and chairs were beige. Even the attendees seemed beige, talking little as they gathered. And I'm certain the others found me beige, too. In spite of the heat of the evening and the lukewarm air-conditioning, I was chill with nerves and dread.

The group facilitator sat on the couch. Two other women, about my age, sat across from her and I sat on a chair facing a younger couple seated to her right.

The facilitator introduced herself and asked us to do the same. Then we each gave a general description of our personal experience with Alzheimer's. With no preamble, no explanation of how support groups work or what we should expect during the evening, the facilitator began with her own story.

Her mother had died with pneumonia a few months before. Alzheimer's didn't cause her sickness, but it complicated her recovery to the point that the daughter could state with confidence it was *Alzheimer's* that killed her mother. She spoke of her relief that her mother was finally whole again and free.

As she spoke, my thoughts astonished me. *And you too*, they shouted to the facilitator. *You're free too! You're whole again, too!* In an instant, I felt deeply jealous of that freedom, not just for my mother, but for myself.

The sudden depth of my emotions shocked me. I was almost sickened by the realization that there, in the beige library, I saw my mother's death as a good thing. Not a new concept, surely, but one I had not allowed myself to acknowledge until that moment. It set off a blinding barrage of guilt and shame. I tried to push my thoughts away and take in what this daughter was saying about her own mother's death. Surely she hadn't been as selfish a daughter as I, not as fixated on her own pain. I hoped the envy didn't show on my face.

As she continued to speak, the facilitator passed around a picture of her mother taken at their last Christmas together. I think my mouth fell open, and I might have gasped. How lovely she looked! Her hair was short and stylish; her nails, painted Christmas red. Her clothes fit a little loose on her small frame, but they sparkled with sequins and the colors of the season. Alzheimer's showed itself only in her empty eyes and vacant smile.

Again my feelings welled up, spilled over into my carefully guarded awareness. How much more competent was this daughter than I! Clearly she had protected her mother. At least from the physical dirt and ugliness of Alzheimer's. What would the moderator think if she saw a picture of my mother? In hindsight, I know everyone in attendance may have benefited if I'd had the courage to speak my thoughts aloud. But I could only sit, shamed and silent, as the picture made its way around the little circle.

Judy arrived just in time to see the picture. She introduced herself to the group as my friend and shot me a look that said, "Okay. The five minutes start now."

What did she think of the pretty little lady in the picture? What did she think of that lady's daughter? Judy knew about the physical indignities Alzheimer's thrust on my mother. And now she would see I obviously hadn't fought the monsters as well as I fancied I had.

By the time I pulled my mind away from guilt and back to the meeting, another woman had shared most of her story. "So I'm desperate for a new caregiver for Mom," she ended. "Anybody have a name you can share?"

While suggestions were made and telephone numbers exchanged, I glanced at my friend. The mug of water she carried constantly at work was tucked under her chair. Somehow, seeing it reassured me. It reminded me there was a world outside this room, with normal people leading normal lives, where decisions had to do with what's for dinner and should I water the lawn or will it rain.

Judy took notes and examined the materials the group leader laid out on a table in front of the couch. I wasn't taking in much information anymore, but I knew I had passed the five-minute mark, and I knew I would stay until the end.

Finally it was my turn to speak. My beige frame of mind had turned white with retreat. I offered only a general description of my circumstances: I became aware of my mother's Alzheimer's a few months ago; my father was determined he could take care of Mom at home; I stepped in to help. I spoke a sentence or two about Mom's lack of cooperation and growing hostility, then closed by saying I knew I would benefit from the help, information, and ideas passed on in this group.

Joan, the woman who spoke after me, identified herself as a nurse. Her weary posture, slumped in one of the beige chairs, belied her strong voice. As she described her mother's illness, Joan's anger took over the room. In addition to Alzheimer's, her mother had recently experienced some sort of respiratory problem. She'd been very ill but she hadn't died, Joan explained, and, in fact, her mom would shortly leave the hospital to return to the nursing facility where she lived.

"Great. That's just great." Joan's hands rose and fell as she spoke, like big wet leaves that had been momentarily lifted by a strong wind, then dropped with a splat to the soggy ground. "It's going to take me forever to get her settled again at the home. My work schedule is shot for the next two weeks."

"The home" sounded like a nice place. The staff there had been concerned when Joan's mother went to the hospital and they were already working with Joan to arrange for the additional care her mother needed. But Joan was angry that she was the only family member available to see to her mom's needs.

Looking back, I recognize her loneliness. Her exhaustion. She was in the right place to express her anger—against Alzheimer's, against her mother, against the respiratory problem that had brought no release but only more problems. But on that night, no one in the circle knew quite what to do with Joan's rage. And so it hung there in the air of the library at the church. Invisible, yet dwarfing all the pictures of faith on the beige walls, and all the books with all their wisdom.

Appalled, and still shocked at my own feelings, I sank back into my metal folding chair.

Leeann, the young woman at the end of the circle, was the last to share her story. She introduced her husband, and explained this was her first time to attend the support group meeting.

"I hope next time I come, I can bring my mom with me. My dad has Alzheimer's, but he'll be fine staying with my husband." She described how her father followed them around, his wife or daughter or son-in-law.

Despite his confusion, Leeann said, "Dad's happy to be home with his family. We're glad Alzheimer's didn't steal his personality. He's always been a gentle man. Now I'm not sure he knows our names or how we fit into his life, but he trusts us. You can see his love when he looks at Mom. He can't say it, but we see it in his face."

With a small smile on his face, Leeann's husband held her hand as she talked. I realized there was less tension in the room now. Leeann spoke with obvious certainty that the problems they encountered in caring for her father had solutions. Among those of us who were starved for hope and encouragement, Leeann was a quiet spring of faith.

She finished her sharing with a question about daycare programs for Alzheimer's patients. She said her mother was also looking into hiring someone to come to their home two or three times a week to help. "Planning for the future," Leeann said.

Planning for the future. That sounded good to me. But I couldn't imagine my father going along with either of the options Leeann's mother was considering.

Judy and I walked to the parking lot. "Well, you did it! How do you feel?" she asked.

I studied her face for some hint of what she expected me to say. How she thought I should feel. I saw no clues. "I don't know. I really don't know. Let me think on it and maybe I'll know tomorrow." We parted with a hug. As I drove home, I realized I'd forgotten to thank her for coming.

When I saw her at work the next day, I made sure to tell her how grateful I was. Then, in an unusual fit of candor, I confessed: the meeting had left me feeling worse, not better.

"Some better," I said, "but more worse. If it hadn't been for Leeann and her husband, I don't think I'd ever go back."

I could see her surprise. "I felt the same way," she said. "It seemed like there just wasn't enough helping to offset all the hurting. So...let's try a different group!"

As I contemplated going to another group, I realized that, while I hadn't enjoyed it, I knew I benefited from the frank talk and the honest expression of emotion from the group members. And as difficult as it was to hear their pain, I was reassured to know I wasn't alone in my anger and grief. In their words, I recognized my own experiences and feelings. I saw that while some caregivers had an easier time than Dad and I, others surely had it harder. I heard about options, other ways that Mom's needs could be met, ways that would give my father and me a rest and maybe even improve Mom's quality of life.

But the miracle of that first support group meeting was that Leeann and her husband decided to make their first visit on the same night I was there. Leeann's quiet spirit touched me. Her proactive approach energized me. Her loving acceptance of her father's condition reassured me that I wasn't living in some unrealistic and unhealthy la-la land of optimism. She and her husband exuded a sense of well-being and faith in the midst of sadness and loss. They were strong, and they made me feel strong.

A couple of weeks later, Judy and I went to a different group meeting. This one met in a large nursing and rehabilitation hospital that housed a unit specifically for Alzheimer's patients. One of the directors of that unit led the group.

The meeting took place in a spacious, attractively furnished parlor area, separated from the main lobby by French doors. Fifteen or twenty people, each wearing a name tag, sat on couches, easy chairs, and straight-backed dining chairs, visiting with each other before the meeting began. Men and women, young and old, some dressed in work attire, some more casually. Cookies and lemonade beckoned from a table to the side of the meeting area.

At one end of the circle of chairs and couches, talking with the people seated closest to her, was a smiling Leeann! We found out later that the older lady beside her, also engaged in eager conversation, was her mother.

The meeting began, and the facilitator invited new members to introduce themselves. After that, conversation moved around the circle. Most people shared their personal experiences and observations, some asked questions, and a few passed on their turn to speak. Whether they came to listen, to pick up ideas, or just to be with others who understood the challenges and pain of being a caregiver for someone with Alzheimer's, I realized that even those who didn't speak added to the circle of care, trust, and understanding at the meeting. Those who did address the group almost always received suggestions, comments, and answers from the group leader as well other attendees.

Most members of the group were sons or daughters of Alzheimer's patients. Others were husbands or wives. Some attendees were related to patients who lived at this particular care facility, but most were not. Some lived with the person they were responsible for; others lived far away. Almost every imaginable Alzheimer's situation was represented.

In the years that followed, I attended many meetings in that parlor. Despite the serious nature of the discussions, the atmosphere remained upbeat. The meetings were not misery-loves-company convocations, but rather two-or-twenty-heads-are-better-than-one sessions. Information was expert; speakers were often invited for special presentations. Suggestions were abundant; sympathy, energy, and hope flowed freely.

Still, I couldn't persuade Dad to come with me or go in my place. Never elaborating on his reasons, he simply said, "Oh, no. I don't think that's for me." I wish he had tried. Maybe he would have received some comfort from listening and sharing. Maybe his single-minded drive and his boundless love for Mom would have provided support for someone else. Maybe he would have been to someone else the miracle Leeann was to me that first night.

As it was, I think he and Mom benefited from my going. The meetings were sometimes difficult, but even then, they were a stepladder for me, a way out of the dark hole of hiding and self-pity and hopelessness. Once I began climbing the ladder, hands reached down to pull me up higher, up to a road we could all travel together. And I found that I could help others, too, in their journey on that road. Eventually, I discovered I could achieve the firmest footing on the path when, with one hand, I accepted the help offered by other travelers, while, with the other, I reached back to help someone else along.

NOTES

> If possible, wade, don't dive into the ocean of Alzheimer's education. I realize now that I went to the first caregivers' conference with unrealistic expectations. I wanted someone to hold my hand and tell me everything would be okay. But all I could hear was the bad news: the relentless nature of the disease and the challenges of caregiving. My pain was so new, I couldn't hear the encouragement being offered, and I didn't see the value of the resources that surrounded me. What I needed was a one-on-one meeting with a professional who could talk to me about Alzheimer's, what we could expect, how we should prepare. And I needed to meet someone who had walked in my shoes and survived. With more knowledge and more time to digest the reality of my parents' situation, I believe I could have gained much more from the conference.

> **I urge you to give support groups a try. Or two.** Use the Five Minute Rule. Even if you're certain no one there will have anything valuable to offer you, consider that you might have invaluable advice, encouragement, or help for someone else.

> The need for someone to stay with your loved one while you attend the meeting can help you start forming the circle of stand-in caregivers who will provide help and respite for you later on.

> An alternative might be to attend a support group that meets in an Alzheimer's care facility. Usually attendees are invited to bring their loved ones to be cared for during the meeting by the staff in a dayroom setting with other Alzheimer's patients. Your local chapter of the Alzheimer's Association can help you locate the group that fits your needs and your schedule.

> Different groups will have different "personalities." Don't hesitate to shop around to find the group where you feel most comfortable.

> Try not to feel shy or self-conscious, at least not for long. The group is for you. It exists to meet your needs, either directly or by giving you information and referrals.

> The power of sharing common experiences is something that can't be described; you have to experience it. I pray you'll give support groups a try.

Let 'Em Eat Meatloaf

I will wait for the Lord....I will put my trust in him.
—ISAIAH 8:17, NIV

The day my parents signed the powers of attorney was the day Dad made German meatloaf. When he told me about it that morning, the meatloaf I mean, I flexed my jaws and swallowed hard, getting in some practice for what I feared would be a really difficult process later that evening. It just seemed impossible that a recipe could call for the addition of sauerkraut to an otherwise okay-sounding meatloaf. The caraway seeds were questionable. But *sauerkraut?*

Dad had been on a meatloaf quest for months, maybe a year. For a while after Mom stopped cooking, my parents dined on frozen dinners. At first it was a novelty to them. Besides, they insisted, the dinners were delicious. I checked out the nutritional information on the side of the red cardboard packages and agreed that the meals were at least as nourishing as the crackers and sardines they used to feast on in my childhood.

During the frozen-dinner era, Mom chose which variety of meal they would heat up. Dad made salad, toasted bread, and set the table. *Voila!* Dinner was served. But eventually the new wore off the deep-dish lasagna and the country fried chicken and the Salisbury steak with vegetables in rich tomato sauce. That's when Dad began his search for the perfect meatloaf.

He started with the standard ingredients: onion, green peppers, tomato sauce, ground beef, maybe some pork. Then he ventured out to mustard, brown sugar, barbecue sauce. He made it Italian, Southern, and Western. He made it Mexican, Texan, and Cajun. Never satisfied, he tweaked each recipe and then began combining them. Southern Italian meatloaf. Texican meatloaf.

The German meatloaf recipe defied tweaking. Mom watched as if hypnotized while Dad assembled the ingredients that morning. Silent, unsmiling, she turned her head from side to side as he strode back and forth across the kitchen—tomatoes, caraway seeds, dill, onion, sauerkraut, mustard. The carefully selected beef waited in the refrigerator. Finally all was in readiness. The ingredients were lined up along the counter in the precise order in which they would be used when Dad assembled the meatloaf later in the day.

While he was preparing for dinner, I was still trying to help my mother through breakfast. I finally persuaded her to drink a bit of orange juice, then brushed her hair and put on her shoes. While I cleared away the dishes, I could hear Dad brushing his teeth. He brushed forever, and then he brushed some more. I knew he was putting off the day's main event, going to the bank to sign the powers of attorney.

I was nervous, too. But when Dad came out of the bathroom, teeth shining, we had no more excuse for delay. When he still didn't say the words, I did. "Well! Okay! Let's head for the bank!"

I had made a trial run to customer service the day before to confirm someone would be available to notarize signatures on the documents. I knew where to sign in, whom to see, where to wait. I had the documents prepared and had explained them to my mother many times. I was prepared to explain them again, if necessary—slowly, clearly, very few words. I knew the less fuss made over their importance, the better.

What I couldn't gauge was what Mom's unsmiling face meant on this particular day. In general, that face didn't bode well for her willingness to cooperate. With each glance in the rearview mirror, I gripped the steering wheel a little tighter and said another prayer that we'd accomplish what we needed to at the bank.

Please let Mom sign the papers, Lord. Let her not scowl at strangers. Let it not be too loud in there, Lord. Noise makes Mom nervous. And if she gets in there and tells us no, if she says she won't sign anything, please help her to just say it, not shout. But please, Lord, let her sign the papers.

Day by day, we were finding it more impossible to predict, anticipate, plan. All I knew to do was pray and trust.

Mom kept quiet until we arrived at the bank…where she announced she would wait for us in the car.

Panic played over Dad's face, but his voice was calm. "Oh, no, baby. We need you to come and help us. Just to sign your name on the papers we talked about."

As he spoke, he moved out of the car. His steps were quick and smooth, as if his feet weren't touching the ground. He opened her door. Offered his hand.

And there it was. Another miracle. With no argument, Mom grasped her purse and looked toward the bank.

"I can do it. I don't need any help!" she snapped as she seized Dad's hand. He and I started breathing again and we all headed into the building.

A lot of people were waiting for the notary. I tried to banish the fear bubbling in my stomach and helped Mom, who still insisted she needed no help, to a seat kindly vacated by a young woman who had watched us approach—Mom in her shamrock tennis shoes, clutching a worn and empty handbag; Dad, jingling the change in his pocket with one hand and holding a manila document folder with the other; me, scanning the scene for signs of potential disaster. I smiled a big thank you for the seat.

Hazards abounded. People talked all around us. Children too young for school played chase through the sitting area, squealing and running around our feet. One little boy stared as Mom lowered herself by infinitesimal degrees to the faded flowers on the sofa cushion. A toddler with a bag of snacks fell and crackers flew everywhere. The chasers crushed them and the baby cried and the bank speaker squawked in our ears.

Names were called and people came and went. Trying to avoid one of the children, someone bumped my knee. I glanced anxiously at Mom—and she smiled at me! Not a grin, but a relaxed little faraway smile. Surely my prayers were being answered. Maybe the worn couch reminded her of home. Or the crowd of children reminded her of days with her brothers and sisters. Whatever the explanation, the longer we waited, the more relaxed she became.

Finally the speaker called Dad's name.

"Let's go, baby!" he bellowed to Mom, and we made our way around a potted plant to the other side of a shoulder-high partition where the notary sat at a desk. Her thin lips formed a tight smile as, with a flash of red fingernails, she gestured toward two straight-backed chairs. Dad sat in one. Mom smiled her serene, faraway smile as she lowered herself into the other.

Dad and the notary exchanged only a few words before he signed his portion of the documents. The red-tipped fingers promptly signed, stamped, and sealed them. But when the notary pushed the papers and pen over toward Mom, the process slowed to a crawl. Mom's hands didn't move. She just looked around, toward my father, toward me, as if expecting something... something. At length, with her eyebrows raised as if in question, Mom met the sharp gaze of the dark-suited woman on the other side of the desk.

"Do you understand what this paper is?" the notary asked. "Do you know that it means your daughter here can handle all your affairs?"

Mom just smiled at her.

"Your daughter could," said the notary, "manage your accounts for you."

Mom kept smiling.

In a patient voice but with a slight frown at me, the notary made one more try. "Do you understand that your daughter could get to all your money?"

Finally leaning forward, Mom slowly and kindly explained the power of attorney to the notary. "Oh, yes, she can get to my money. She can do everything Daddy can. In case I need help. Right, Daddy?" She glanced at my father then looked back to the notary.

During a long moment, no one moved or spoke. Outside the cubicle even the laughing children seemed to have gone silent. At last the notary told Mom she could sign right there on that line beside the yellow mark. I watched as she handed Mom the red and blue ballpoint pen with the bank logo on the side.

I had thought that with the questions asked and answered, I needn't worry what would happen next. But watching Mom take the pen from the red-tipped fingers, I realized I was wrong. She held it clumsily, a far cry from the elegant grasp I had worked as a child to imitate. While she studied the pen, I prayed. I prayed, not that Mom would remember how to sign her name, but that I wouldn't see that look on her face. The look she routinely gave me when the doctor asked her what year it was, who was the president, what were those three words he had asked her to remember. That look that said, "Please tell me what to do."

I continued to pray, and Mom continued to study the pen. The paper. Her fingers. Her mouth moved and she shifted in her chair. She cleared her throat and put her hand to the paper, lifted the pen and twirled it slowly. Then with a look of dreadful concentration, she began to sign her name. Like a butterfly hovering over a flower, lighting, rising, lighting, fluttering, unsteady and delicate and impossibly fragile, her hand guided the pen to form web-thin marks that spelled her name. Miraculously, the name she hadn't signed in more than a year appeared like a ripple on the paper pond. Even today I cannot bear to look at that signature.

"Well, all *right!* Good job, baby!" Dad's voice was much too loud, as usual, but Mom beamed at him, grinning, I imagined, with joy at having pleased him.

The notary did her stamping and sealing, and while Dad gathered the documents, I gathered Mom to leave. The next customer's name had been called and we were walking away from the desk when suddenly Mom turned. She pulled her arm from my grasp and shuffled back toward the notary. I felt the blood rushing to my face.

The notary came around from behind her desk to meet Mom, who took her hand and leaned in close to her face.

"Thank you so much," Mom said to the notary in a barely audible voice. "We had a lovely time!" With a pat to the red-tipped fingers, she turned back to me and grinned again. It was a feast of smiling, a bounty of miracles.

That night my husband and I arrived at my parents' house just as Dad was putting the meatloaf in the oven. While it cooked, we all sat at the table and talked, our conversation interspersed with comments on the aromas wafting from the kitchen. I had decided it was wise to let my husband be surprised with the evening's menu, but at last we made him try to guess what new and startling variation characterized this latest meatloaf. Of course, there was no way he could anticipate that someone, somewhere, had come up with the idea of putting sauerkraut and caraway seeds into this classic of American cooking. When Dad could stand it no longer, he made the great announcement: tonight we would dine on German meatloaf. "With sauerkraut!"

And so we did. Three of us pronounced it quite "different." Tasty. Moist. Mom fed hers to Charley-Dog, bite by bite, from her own fork. I thought I saw my husband drop Charley a bite or two as well.

Over coffee and ice cream, we agreed it was a very special meatloaf indeed. Fitting for this day on which so much was accomplished, this night when we had so much to be grateful for. The legal process I had dreaded, that had seemed so cold and impersonal and impossible, was now like a net stretched wide and strong beneath the high, unstable bridge we were crossing. Mom had once again seen my father's pride shine out to her, and Dad and I had seen joy light her face and lighten her steps.

And there was also that great and comforting truth that filled the room around us. No one spoke it; no one needed to. We simply knew—my husband, my father, and I—we knew, and rejoiced: we would never have to eat German meatloaf again.

NOTES

> The need to attend to legal matters early on cannot be overemphasized. Legal documents must be signed before your loved one's condition progresses to the point at which he or she is no longer capable of understanding them.

> Though there are many documents that may apply to your loved one's situation. Three in particular are usually mentioned as necessary in the case of someone with Alzheimer's:
> 1. A will.
> 2. A living will, having to do with end-of-life healthcare issues.
> 3. A durable power of attorney, one that remains valid when the person no longer has the capacity to make decisions regarding his/her own needs.

> Be aware: Laws vary from state to state. You will need legal advice specific to the state where your loved one resides. The Alzheimer's Association, your local Area Agency on Aging, and other organizations that focus on needs of the older population can help direct you to the information you need.

On Maneuvers

Our God....we have no power to face this vast army....We
do not know what to do, but our eyes are on you.
—2 CHRONICLES 20:12, NIV

Two things about Mom's hygiene never ceased to amaze me. One was that her constitution could tolerate so much dirt with no obvious adverse effects. The other was Dad's endless optimism in this as in all issues surrounding my mother.

Some mornings I arrived to be greeted by Dad's broad smile and proud proclamation that Mom had gone to the bathroom already.

Alone.

"And look! She's eating her toast and drinking her juice— how 'bout some more plum jam, baby?"

With a smile smeared like jelly across my face, I'd rush to clean what I feared was not plum jam from her fingers and her nails. Dad's bad eyesight protected him from some disgusting realities. My love for him kept me from saying the words I should have shouted: *"You have to clean her hands, Daddy! Don't you see how nasty they are? No, I guess you can't see it, but you have to clean her hands for her. Every time! They always need it! Eating with her fingers, with those filthy fingers—she's going to get sick!"*

How could I not have said that? But I didn't. And, miraculously, Mom never got sick. Never a skin rash, an infection, nothing.

As for Dad's optimism, it simply never waned. For example, he was certain he could *talk* Mom into the bathtub. "How 'bout a good ole' bath today, honey? Oh boy, that'll feel good!"

The truth was that his cajoling did as much harm as good.

As demons are prone to do, the demons of Alzheimer's homed in on the traits of my mother's personality that were already hard to live with, and exaggerated them. The good days became fewer, and on the bad days, we dealt with the extremes. Mom's reluctance to take direction became absolute willfulness. Her suspicious nature became cold meanness. Her fears became paranoia. And her ever-casual attitude toward bathing, probably formed during her childhood when bathing eleven children was less important than feeding and clothing them, became a determination to avoid it at all costs.

Mom turned Dad's encouraging words back on him with sarcasm and ridicule. "Oh, the big man thinks I need a bath! It'll make me feel good! You take a bath, big man! You feel good! I don't need it."

Intellectually I knew the struggle against dirt was also a struggle against her confusion and fear, but as each day grated harder against the surface of my emotions, I found myself thinking that Mom said no to bathing because she *could*. She could sit and refuse to go into the bathroom. She could stiffen and refuse to get undressed. She could make it hard for us. Very hard. Simply by saying no.

She said it quickly, even though her mind worked slowly. She said it with utter finality, even though confusion ruled her life. How did she do that? Willfulness? Again and again I had to remind myself that Mom was no longer capable of being willful.

And as I accepted that, I came up with a more plausible explanation. Mom's "no" was instinctive. It was born of her instinct to survive.

With patience and perspective that could only come from the Lord, I began to understand. For someone who sometimes had trouble remembering things as basic as how to go from standing to sitting, the many moves required to take off a blouse and pants had to be confusing and exhausting. For someone unable to find her bed every night and the kitchen every morning, going into a shower stall once a week was foreign and frightening.

Mom's greatest comfort consisted of sitting in one position in her straight-backed dining chair at the kitchen table. She obviously saw no benefit in moving around. Besides, brushing teeth, trimming nails, washing hair, and bathing required a lot of close contact—a great loss of her privacy. Mom couldn't name the good feelings she was losing, but she made it clear: losing them felt bad.

In the special Alzheimer's units in some nursing homes, the door to each client's room holds a picture of the person who lives there, as that person appeared before he or she was robbed of self by Alzheimer's. What exquisite statements those pictures make!

"The person in this room is as real as you or me. He had electric-blue eyes, not the clouded, suspicious ones you see today. He danced with his wife and read the New York Times. Now he doesn't understand the world he used to command. He remembers few people, comprehends little, reads not at all. But he is real."

On another door, the picture says, "She used to dress like the models in fashion magazines. She played golf and rode horses. Now she's afraid to move far or fast. She's not *as* she was, but she's still *who* she was. You think you're seeing her, but today you're seeing mostly Alzheimer's."

I wish we had displayed more pictures of Mom. I wish we had reminded family and visitors of her beauty and personality.

And we needed to remind ourselves. *I* needed to remember. Virtually every one of Mom's physical features was marked by the graffiti of Alzheimer's: scaly skin, matted hair, tobacco-stained fingernails. Old, worn clothes dotted with cigarette burns. Tennis shoes worn to an even shade of dirty, with rubber soles separated at the heels. Stained dentures, crusty eyelids, glazed eyes.

She looked like a skeleton in camouflage.

Just maintaining some minimal standard of cleanliness consumed enormous amounts of my patience and energy. Dad tried to help. But his effort consisted of words: *encouraging* Mom to bathe. It was up to me to remove the dirt.

The division of labor resulted in large part from the obvious difference in our purposes. Dad's primary goal was to maintain their status as a couple, to see to it that the two of them could live together for as long as possible. And my job, as I saw it at the time, was to keep each of them alive. Dad had the nights, dark and scary. I had the days, glaring and wild. At night, they slept together in the same bed. During the day, they lived as well as they could. Together. And I helped.

But I felt alone. Many times, I know, Dad saw me as a necessary evil. One of those times was when I insisted that, willing or not, Mom must bathe. In order to preserve peace, Dad usually just gave up when she refused a bath. I suppose he saw bathing as one of many things not necessary to their life together. Doctor's appointments, taking medication, eating—those things were necessary. Bathing, shampooing, and clean clothes were not. Trimmed fingernails and toenails were not. Clean hands and face were not. Dad saw those things as desirable, but not worth fighting for.

So I did the fighting.

Strategy was required. Creativity, surely, but also strategy on the order of a military campaign. Ambush. I learned that action taken with no prior warning overcame many obstacles in many different situations. And working *with* Mom's negative tendencies, instead of against them, proved effective.

The first part of the plan was to pick a day when Mom had already had some exercise. Her muscles were warmed up a bit but tired, making her likelier to cooperate than to fight.

I prepared everything in advance—and in secret. Soap, shampoo, towel, washcloth. Shower chair in place. Clean clothes at hand.

Then, after a flurry of winking at Dad behind Mom's back, I'd take her arm in a conspiratorial manner. "Let's go in here," I'd whisper, my face close to hers, my finger to my lips in a sign of secrecy.

To my father's "What are you girls up to?" I replied, "That's for us to know and you to find out," as I grinned sideways at my mother. Often this elicited a broad smile that let me know she'd shuffle off with me wherever I led her.

Once in the bathroom, I continued the conspiracy with theatrical whispering. "Daddy doesn't need to know everything we're doing! This is the girls' time, right? Here, have a seat right here and I'll help you."

Confused, but pleased to be "tricking" my father, she sat on the commode as I indicated, perched on the edge of the lid. While she sat, I talked nonstop and undressed her.

Once we started removing her clothes, it seemed Mom's confusion as to what was taking place made her powerless to fight with anything other than words, if she fought at all. My slow but non-stop movements and my constant stream of softly spoken words seemed to keep her attention on the immediate experience, giving her no opportunity to worry about what might happen next. She appeared calmed, entranced even, by the fact that all my attention was focused on her.

"Here, let me help you into the tub," I'd say, always holding her arm. I acted with every expectation of her complete cooperation, speaking and moving as though this were a prearranged plan we were executing together.

I eased her into the bathtub, holding her arm with one hand, helping her lift her feet over the edge with the other. Talking, always talking. The bath chair was ready at the far end of the tub, the warm water already running gently from the handheld showerhead which lay on the bottom of the tub, pointing down.

So there we were. Mom sitting on a little white chair, her eyes darting in every direction, looking ready to jump out of her skin, which was, of course, all she was wearing at the moment. And me at her side, bending over her, talking and feeling victorious that we had made it this far.

"Here—you must be a little cold, Mama," I'd say with great solicitude, directing the warm spray slowly upward from her feet to her legs to her arms and back.

She sat up straighter as the stream of water moved higher. "Oh, thank you, child."

Quickly now, because she really did get chilled easily, I'd put soap on a washcloth and bathe her. I tried at first to let her do the washing, but her grip on the cloth was so uncertain that it barely touched her skin. As time passed, I saw she had no idea what to do with the warm, bubbly cloth. So I washed her, talking quietly all the while. I gave the play-by-play of the bathing action, speculated on Dad's frustration at not knowing what we were up to, predicted his surprise when we returned to the table.

I could see her relax under the warm spray. Sitting on this chair was not so different from sitting in her chair at the table. I kept her attention with my words and my slow but steady movements.

But when the time came to wash her hair, the relaxing was over.

First came the discussion. As I moved the water up toward her head, I said some sentence with "shampoo" in it. She reacted as if I had said, "Let's decapitate you."

"No, no, don't do that!"

"It'll just take a second or two. Here we go...."

"No! Please! You might get my hair wet."

"It'll feel so good to have clean hair, Mama."

"I just washed it yesterday."

"Well, let's do it with this nice new shampoo." At that point, she'd struggle to stand up. "No, no, I don't like it. I don't want to."

Even when she didn't fight, it wasn't easy. Mom couldn't understand instructions to tilt her head back so the water would flow away from her face. I needed the dexterity of an octopus to hold a washcloth over her eyes, wet her hair, and put a little shampoo on it, all the while staying ready to steady her in the chair if she started leaning.

Her matted waves were surely not attractive, but the hair itself hid a scalp covered with scales and flakes, impossible to remove even with my gentle but ardent scrubbing. So we did the best we could. I skipped hair washing only in the direst emergencies—usually, the times when she began waving her arms and shouting when I said the shampoo sentence.

Then one day, without even thinking about it, I conducted a Hair Washing Operation with the same stealth I used for the overall Bath Campaign. No flag waving, no fife and drum corps, no "Shampoo!" battle cry.

Instead, *ambush* again. Gentle, to be sure, but very effective, I found. Once Mom was in the tub, the surprise shampoo technique worked almost every time.

The process began with the "one last rinse" of her back. I inched the spray to the back of her neck and then to the back of her head. From there, I moved it quickly to the top. I used my free hand to shield her ears and then her face. I laid the showerhead in the bottom of the tub, and, with both hands free, squeezed out some shampoo and gave her head a fast ten-second scrub.

I'm not sure why I had thought I must announce every action I was about to take. Most activities went more smoothly when I didn't. There were times when I needed Mom to know because I needed her help, but shampooing wasn't one of those times. I was confident I could get it done. My confidence probably kept *her* calmer also. And while she worked to understand the unexpected sensation of water on her head, she was less likely to fear—or fight—what might come next.

I never stopped talking to her, softly talking: "Oh, I really like this shower thing Daddy got for you. It makes everything so easy and comfortable. Mmmm…don't you like the smell of this new shampoo? Well, my goodness! Let me give you this cloth to hold over your eyes. Here—hold it just like this—yes! Perfect! Now we can just rinse this all off and we'll be through. Oh, Mama! Your hair will just shine. I think it's shining already! Okay, let me get a towel around your shoulders.…"

Now bath time was almost finished. One towel around her shoulders kept her warm as I dried her hair with another. I helped her out of the tub and let her sit on a towel on the lid of the commode. Mom was cold in all seasons of the year, even when I was sweating, so I put her clean clothes on as quickly as possible.

First her shirt, then, as she still sat, her underwear and slacks. These I would pull up only as far as her knees. I brushed her wet hair as she continued to rest from the extreme exertion of the whole process. Finally I'd help her stand and, with her hands on my back or shoulder, I'd bend to pull her underwear and slacks up to her waist.

"Oh, Mama! Just look! Here in this mirror. You look so nice! And look! Your hair is just beautiful."

Winter or summer, we never dried her hair with a hair dryer. I knew the sound and the blowing would be too much for her to tolerate after the protracted confusion and activity of her bath. Standing before the mirror, my hand under her elbow, she smiled at her reflection, a small, wondering smile. I looked in the mirror and saw the miracle: my mother.

"Let's go surprise Daddy!" I'd whisper, and she would turn to me and grin.

With great drama, I called out to Dad. "Here we come, Daddy! Close your eyes! We have a surprise for you!" My words echoed merrily off the pink tile that covered the walls and floor.

"Hurry up, child!" Mom was already padding down the hall.

"Okay! You can open your eyes now!" My voice, still artificially loud, signaled the beginning of a long stream of compliments from my father. Without a word, Mom basked in them, perhaps patting her head or pulling at her shirt to let my father know he'd not yet mentioned her clean hair or the blouse that was "brand new" each time she wore it.

How often did we go through this bathing drill? Once a week, I would like to say. In truth, it was more like once a month. Definitely not a healthy situation. Because of her illness, Mom got dirty. Head-to-toe dirty, every day. But we did the best we could at the time. The bathing process was mentally and physically exhausting for her. Besides, "surprising" her that often would have done her, and thus all of us, more harm than the good we gained through her cleanliness.

A solution, of course, would have been professional help. My reluctance to force Dad to hire someone to take care of Mom's physical needs could have had dire results. Her lack of hygiene could have led to an illness that separated them from each other for a long time. But by some blessing, her hair, scalp, and skin tolerated the dirt well. She never had an upset stomach or an infected wound, not even a rash.

I know now that I should have tried harder to make Dad accept outside help. In addition to the benefits it might have brought to the quality of my parents' lives, my own family deserved it. My parents' "independence" resulted in an unhealthy burden on me and therefore on my family. But I dreaded imposing my will on my father. I imagined he might see it as a final blow to his status as my mother's spouse and protector. The truth, of course, is that he was not independent. And the irony is that accepting professional help would have increased, not decreased, his freedom.

As it was, bath days required a huge expenditure of energy, creativity, and patience. But the obvious feeling of satisfaction we shared at the end of bath day was sufficient reward. Happiness lit Mom's face when she looked at herself in the mirror. And when Dad opened his eyes to her, his surprise was not to find her still so beautiful, but only to see her sparkling clean. She was never less than beautiful to him. When he looked at Mom, Dad's eyesight never failed him.

NOTES

> For those with Alzheimer's, inattention to personal hygiene usually becomes an aversion to it. In my mother's case, that aversion became so strong that often the bath or shower I had planned for her turned into nothing more than a warm washcloth on her face and hands. You may have to make similar adjustments to your standards of cleanliness. It's hard to accept, but good to remember: health is the goal, not appearance. Your doctor can tell you if your loved one's health is suffering due to lack of hygiene.

> When you begin an activity that may be met with resistance, announcing your intentions and seeking your loved one's cooperation may not be the easiest ways to accomplish your task. For me, just *doing it* was usually the best strategy. I used whatever story was necessary to get Mom to the required location—the bathroom, for instance—and then, without explanation or question, I started *doing* what we were there for.

> In stressful situations, my nonstop talking seemed to both calm and distract Mom.

> Getting advice on bathroom safety equipment will help both you and your loved one feel safer in the bathroom. You can visit a medical equipment shop in person or explore your options with help from the Alzheimer's Association or community senior health organizations. Handrails, a shower chair, and special mats for the floor are some of the items you'll need. Putting them in place before they're needed may lessen your loved one's confusion later on when using them is absolutely necessary.

> Help with bathing and shampooing is another area where, I believe, getting professional help is worth whatever effort is required. The issues of health and safety cannot be overstated. Though I managed with Mom, a professional could almost certainly have handled bath day faster, better, and more safely.

It's Okay

The Lord watches over you— the Lord is your shade at your right hand; the sun will not harm you by day, nor the moon by night. The Lord will keep you from all harm—he will watch over your life; the Lord will watch over your coming and going both now and forevermore.

—PSALM 121:5–8, NIV

I recall watching on television the ceremonies surrounding the burial of President Ronald Reagan.

At one point, red and white stripes of sturdy woven fabric filled the television screen. The camera held the tight shot for several impossibly long seconds, until a hand moved into the picture. Fingers brushed across the fabric, rippled over the seams. As microphones picked up music playing in the background, at last the camera retreated, revealing Nancy Reagan standing by her husband's flag-draped coffin. Her shoulders were slightly rounded, her hand extended, her eyes cast down to where she touched the flag. Her lips were turned up—almost, but not quite, smiling. The very public nature of the event seemed lost on her.

Bending close to the red and white stripes, she spoke. Just a couple of words, it appeared to me. A couple of words, a little pat on the flag, and then she squared her shoulders and rejoined the public scene.

What did she say? The microphones gave viewers only music, but I have a guess. I think she told him, "It's okay." One last time.

How many hundreds of times might she have said that to him

during his illness? How many hundreds of times did Dad and I say those words to my mother? Ronald Reagan, husband, father, former president of the United States. Marie Bailey, wife, mother, former can-do woman. Two disparate people who shared the terrible connection of Alzheimer's. Losing touch with any sense of the familiar, day by relentless day.

"It's okay. It's okay." Did they ever believe us? Sometimes, I think. Sometimes my mother did.

* * *

Before Alzheimer's, the evening hours were special to my parents. They sat at their kitchen table, half-watching the news on television, half-reviewing their day. Back then, the kitchen was filled with smoke from Mom's cigarette. They didn't care. The tablecloth was worn, with ashes strewn across it. They didn't mind; they'd buy another when they found a pattern they liked. Laughing at their own stories, they'd miss the weather report and ask each other about it and be irritated and get over it.

The pleasantness of evening they held so precious was one of the last remnants of their daily lives to go irrevocably wrong. It had a long way to fall and it fell slowly, like petals dropping. As Alzheimer's ate past the corners and into the heart of their lives, the banter, remembering, and laughter were replaced by Mom's hostility and repeated questions.

Before the light could fade outside the window by her chair, she would tell my father or me to close the blinds. We complied in silence and sat with her in the darkness, listening to news of the world in this room that too quickly assumed the flickering dimensions and absurdity of the TV screen.

Sooner or later, Mom would ask...something. The question *du soir*.

"Where did this come from?"

"What, baby? Where did *what* come from?" Dad answered her.

She hit her hand flat on the table. "What is this thing?"

"Oh! It's our new tablecloth! Isn't it fine?"

"I don't like it."

"But, baby, you picked it out!"

"No, I didn't. It's ugly."

"We got it at the store the other day. They had a bunch of them. You liked this one."

"A bunch of what? What is this thing? I don't like it."

"A tablecloth. You liked it yesterday!"

Picking at the fresh folds of the cloth, Mom would begin again. "No, really, come on. What is this thing?"

Her anger and fear played out in endless variations. Sweet memories were replaced by nightmare scenarios she relived again and again. A weather report she heard on television became a disaster of my father's making. She was certain I had wrecked the pickup truck the news pictured on the freeway. Everything she saw and heard became fodder for her fears. Or her anger. Or both.

"What did that man say?" she might ask Dad.

"The guy on TV? He said to be sure to lock your car while you do your Christmas shopping."

"Where is our car? Is it locked?"

"It's in the garage, baby."

Mom started rocking back and forth in her chair. "Is that outside?"

"Right outside the door."

"It's outside? The car. Where is the car?"

Sighing, Dad switched TV stations. "It's okay. It's all locked up."

"Oh, come *on*.... Where?"

"In the garage, where we always keep it."

"Is it locked?"

"Yes. It's okay. It's wonderful. All locked up in the garage."

Mom shouted this time. "But where is the car? Did they take it?"

"The car is safe. No one can take it."

"Is it locked?"

Sometimes I stepped in, trying to reassure her with a different viewpoint. Or, even better, change the subject altogether. But I found more success by *taking action* to alleviate her fear. Irrational fear, yes, but real fear, nonetheless.

Moving toward the door, I might say, "I'll go check on it right away. Thank you for reminding me, Mama." Then I went outside, stayed a minute, came back inside, and told her, "Yes. I saw the car. It's safe."

That might be the end of it. Or we might begin again.

I tried to imagine her view of the situation. How unsettling would I find it to look down and see something I couldn't put a name to? Especially if many of my belongings were spread across this thing—my lunch plate, my cigarettes, my favorite ashtray. How maddening would it be to hear the person I trust most in the whole frightening world "lie" to me and tell me I had chosen this foreign object? How frustrated would I be at having no help at all in keeping the car safe? I tried to imagine her feelings and I was too successful.

But that was usually as I was driving home, hours later. In the moment, while I sat with her and Dad and listened to her questions, my only goal was to convince her everything was okay. Pat her hand, hold her long fingers in my short, square ones and tell her, "It's okay, Mama. We have it all taken care of."

She almost always responded with a look of confusion. Then more questions.

But *sometimes....* Sometimes her frozen face would thaw and melt, the brittle arches of fear becoming warm wrinkles of trust as she relaxed in the semidarkness.

Other times, the icy hardness would break with explosive energy. She would call us names and inform us she was smarter than we thought and we couldn't fool her. On those evenings, Dad and I looked at each other through the cigarette smoke, dreading what might happen next.

Mom's anger, always acidic, had grown more unreasonable with the onset of Alzheimer's. Meaner. A powerful manifestation of her fear, it threatened to become uncontrollable. At times, our only reassurance that she wouldn't harm us or herself was our certainty that we were physically stronger than she.

But the miracle was that we were never driven by Alzheimer's to the limit of our strength. Experience told us even the worst evenings could end well. Somehow, by bedtime it would be okay.

Hours ticked away as the dusky window by Mom's chair grew darker. Cigarette after cigarette smoldered in the ashtray while she either kept a stubborn silence or found halting but passionate ways to use all our family's forbidden words. Not just the common four-letter words, but the ones on our family list: shut up, pee, stink. She could use them effectively, in proper syntax, for almost the entire duration of her illness. They hit Dad's face like spit.

Worst of all were the nights when Mom wished she were dead.

"I wish I could just die. I'd rather be dead than here!"

Dad would turn, put both elbows on the table, and drop his head. Mom, in the cold light thrown by television images, rocking in her chair and shuffling her feet, would intone a chant of wishing she were dead while Dad shook his head to the cadence. I could only watch, looking first at Mom's wrinkled face and uncombed hair, then at Dad's square fingers clenched over the top of his head.

There we sat. Collectively wounded—gravely, almost mortally wounded—by Alzheimer's.

But Dad and I could fight it yet, and sooner or later, one of us would rally again to the battle. One of us could eventually say "It'll be okay, Mama," and the other would believe.

We said "It's okay" to my mother. We said it for her. And we said it to each other. "It's okay" meant please don't be scared and let's try again. It meant I love you and God loves all of us and we can make things better. It pleaded don't give up. It promised you won't be alone.

"It's okay," patting Mom's tired, shuffling leg. "It's all right," gripping Dad's shoulders tightly. "Let's eat," and one of us would get some chips for Mom and a treat for her to feed the dog before we began pulling dinner from the cabinets and freezer.

Some nights the anger dragged on and Mom refused to eat. Or she fed all her food to Charley-Dog. But somehow things got better for my father and me. Grace and renewed strength smoothed our spirits and patted our despairing hearts and bid us try again. Keep trying. As ugly as Alzheimer's looked and sounded to us from the outside, the monstrosity of experiencing it from the inside was Mom's to bear. If we didn't help, she would die. No one had to tell us that.

As Dad's exhaustion became all too easy to see—his eyes red with fatigue and strain; his body inert, heavy—Mom had finally become very interested in the television. I had to smile at her sudden concentration.

She didn't—couldn't—follow any storyline. But something, something utterly unpredictable, would catch her eye.

"Look at that man, child," she would say to me. "Doesn't he have pretty teeth?"

"Oh, yes, Mama. Beautiful!" I grinned, close to laughing at this indication that she was feeling better. For now. No fear for now. No anger or pain. Just pleasure at seeing someone's teeth on TV and apparent delight at finding the words to comment on them.

Eventually, though, bedtime came. Sometimes welcome, often not.

"I'm not tired."

"It's okay, Mama. Let's just get ready. Then when you *are* tired, you can just go crawl under the covers."

"I'm ready right now. And I'm not tired."

So, time for the ultimate strategy, the same one I employed on bath days. The irresistible force which could almost always move my well-nigh immovable mother.

I would stand up, turn to my father, and, whether he was awake or not, say with dramatic volume, "We'll be back, Daddy. You stay right here. We don't need you to come with us."

Then, turning back to Mom, I'd wink several times, extend my arm to her, and say, "Mama, I need to show you something back here in the other room."

Two women headed for the bathroom to share secrets. It was indeed okay.

By the time we reached the bathroom, Mom had usually forgotten why we were there. But I trusted the familiarity of our ritual to overcome any leftover reluctance. I continued talking in a loud whisper about anything at all, it didn't matter what, as long as I kept repeating that it was talk "just for us girls." All through the difficult clean-up jobs, the persuasion to change her clothes from the skin out, the washing of hands and face—girl talk.

Silliness. "Remember, Mama, how Sis and I used to…."

Or very serious seeking of advice: "I think it's okay to wear flats to a wedding, don't you?"

Non sequiturs were the order of the night. It just didn't matter. It was okay.

At length, with Mom clean and ready for sleep, we walked arm in arm to her side of the bed. Each night we walked past the large black and white portrait of my sister and me. We passed Dad's closet, neat, perfectly arranged, the shoe-shine basket front and center on the top shelf. We passed the chair that held the turquoise and white package of underwear—disposable underwear, ladies' size medium.

We rounded the end of the bed and Mom ran her hand along the wooden rail Dad had attached to the wall to help her steady herself. Always she commented on this, in the same words she used to tell me about the rail on the back porch: "Isn't this nice? Your father made this for me. It's new. Don't you like it?"

I did. I always liked it.

Finally we were in place. "Okay, Mama, just sit down right here."

After rearranging her feet, looking at the bed, and saying "okay" a couple of times, Mom perched on the tiniest edge of the mattress.

"Good, Mama, but let's sit way back. We don't want you falling out of bed!" I would laugh.

She'd look up and say, "Oh, child, what am I thinking? I'm sorry." And then she would stand with difficulty, reposition herself, and sit down again in precisely the same spot.

"Okay, Mama, let's try it again." And we did. If it was just too hard for her that night, I'd virtually pick her up and put her in a safe position, sliding her stiff legs up, helping her straighten them, patting and smoothing and smiling and saying, "There! How's that? Okay?"

Then my reward. The reward for this long evening, this sweet or difficult evening. The reward that made it all okay—these months, these years of saying good-bye. The reward that still consoles, comforts, wraps me in memories of mother and child and child and mother. The reward.

I can hear her yet. "Oh, that's fine, child," Mom tells me with a smile like soft sunlight. "That's really fine. Thank you so much, child. I just don't know what I'd do without you."

"Well, you don't ever have to worry about that, Mama. I'll be here."

I'd bend down, so far down, and kiss her cheek that still smelled of cigarettes and soap, while she closed her eyes, the sunshine smile setting on her face. "Child." Did she remember my name? It didn't matter. I think she knew I was hers. That made everything okay.

NOTES

> Bedtime was the second most difficult time of day for my mother.

> It's worse than useless to argue with someone who has Alzheimer's. Trying to convince Mom of what was clear and obvious to me usually only increased her confusion and/or anger. The better method was to begin with *her* reality. ***Act on the information or situation that your loved one believes to be true.***

> Visible actions work better than words to calm fears. For example, going outside to look at the car worked better than simply assuring Mom it was in the garage.

> Old routines can be helpful, even if they've been absent for a while. For example, the body movements and language associated with going off to another room for girl talk seemed familiar to Mom on some level. She seemed to find them reassuring.

> The distraction of talk often helped me maneuver Mom physically into places she might otherwise have been reluctant to go. I didn't ask her to go or direct her to go. I simply led her in the desired direction with my arm and the bulk of my body, while talking about a totally unrelated subject.

> Even the worst days can turn sweet. *Believing that is essential.* Remembering it can supply a last burst of energy and patience at the end of a day.

Breaking the Fall

*"Though the mountains be shaken and the hills be removed, yet
my unfailing love for you will not be shaken nor my covenant of
peace be removed," says the Lord, who has compassion on you.*
—ISAIAH 54:10, NIV

The muggy atmosphere, even this early in the morning, was typical of mid-June. It pressed against me as I walked to the front porch of my parents' home. The air inside was even worse. Cooler, but damp. Suffocating.

I knew immediately it was not a good day.

"We're back here, Katrinka." Dad's tone and volume told me he was frustrated in the extreme. More than frustrated. Angry? Whatever it was, it was intense and I trotted across the dark shag carpet. Past Mom's stained sofa, past the morning show on the television, down the hall to the doorway of their bedroom.

Mom's morning smell was overpowering. Dad, breathing hard, bent over her where she lay on the floor at the end of their bed. She was on her side, almost but not quite prone, supporting herself with one elbow. Dad, with one hand under her right shoulder, straddled her at her knees. Mom smiled when she saw me, as if she was lying on the beach and I had walked up with two glasses of lemonade in my hands.

I can't remember now why I went to their house that morning. Evenings had become so much more difficult for Dad that I had taken to starting work very early and going to their house shortly after noon.

But on this day, for some forgotten but no less miraculous reason, I decided to make two visits, one early, one later.

I'm sure I drove the familiar route that morning with the too-familiar weight on my chest, the mixture of determination and dread that pulled me with heavy steps day after day into the pink brick house that always reeked of fresh urine and stale cigarettes.

Once inside, things would get better, I knew; they always did. "Better" because I walked into a good day and laughed with relief and gratitude, or "better" because I walked into a bad day but was able to help. Still, each time I stood on the porch announcing my entry with the high-pitched "Yoo-hoo!" our family always used, I was increasingly conscious of the yawning gap between the cheery sound of my voice and the leaden weight of my heart.

Now I stared at the scene at the foot of the bed.

"She fell," Dad said, with the sing-song intonation that told me he was completely outdone with my mother. "She says she can't get up. Marie, please get up! At least help a little!"

Mom looked to him with the same smile she'd given me. "I can't, Daddy," she answered.

"Wait, Daddy—what are you trying to do?" I asked, though it must have been only to give my brain a half second to think. I was certain he planned to help her sit on the bed a step or two from where she lay. "Let me get a chair," I continued before he had a chance to answer.

I stepped over Mom and, from the other side of the room, pulled a straight-backed chair toward her. I also grabbed fresh underwear from the stack beside the bed.

With the chair as close to her as possible, Dad and I lifted Mom upright from beneath her arms. She bore a little of her own weight but tried to sit down immediately.

"Can you hold her up just a second, Daddy?" I was staring at the soaked spot on the carpet. "Just *one* second...."

In a flash, I had removed the overnight underwear and, with little need of her cooperation, I replaced it with a dry pair. Dad let her sink to the chair; she was on the very edge of it, unsteady, looking dazed but still smiling.

"Oh, thank you, Daddy," Mom whispered. "Thank you, child. That's better."

"Can you come in here and have some breakfast?" Dad's voice was full of the same relief that suffused his face.

"Wait, Daddy," I said again. "Just let her sit there for a minute. Don't let go. Mama, I'll get you some juice."

With Dad steadying her, she sipped the orange juice I brought. Between sips, I slipped her gown up over her head and replaced it with a dry t-shirt. *Now we're all feeling better,* I thought.

But when the juice was gone and we helped her stand, she sat again immediately. "I can't do it." That's all she said.

"Does something hurt, Mama? Where do you hurt?" I bent to look in her eyes.

"No, child. I can't."

We tried again. She sank again.

"I can't," she repeated.

"Well you can't stay here all day!" Exasperation and fatigue fought for center stage on Dad's face. "Try again, please."

We lifted; she stood; she sank. This time she said nothing.

Dad and I had been in this spot many times before. Well, not this exact spot, but this predicament. On her sofa, in a restaurant, at the doctor's office, at the breakfast table: Mom "couldn't." Sometimes she couldn't sit. Sometimes she couldn't stand. Sometimes she could stand but not walk. We never knew when a new inability would strike. Or when an old one would return.

Sudden inabilities were part of the heavy sack of dread Dad and I dragged around as we cared for Mom. We never spoke of it; in fact, we pretended it didn't exist. But more and more often now I saw the slump of Dad's shoulders from the weight of that ugly sack, and I felt it more myself from one "yoo-hoo" day to the next.

The predicament was maddening. Dad and I had such a difficult time believing Mom's inabilities were real. We knew her intentional uncooperative streak as a fact of life. Dad had married it; I had grown up with it. Did Alzheimer's rob her of all intentionality? Of all ability to act a certain way to accomplish a certain goal? Eventually it would, we knew, but had she reached that point? Or was she acting out of some habit that her diseased brain belched out at odd moments on random days? Did the sticky tangles that destroyed her mental capabilities also short-circuit her physical abilities—unpredictably, temporarily, repeatedly?

I told myself that when Mom said she couldn't, she really couldn't. But unless I put my fingers in my thoughts so I couldn't hear them, I heard a voice inside me say "I bet she really could."

Now I stood looking at the bedraggled figure in the chair. "You want to just stay in here, Mama?" I asked her. The edge in my voice didn't appear to register with her; with her smile gone, her face was now perfectly expressionless.

Dad sighed. "Sometimes she just goes back to bed. Do you want to go back to bed, baby?"

Mom looked at the bed. "Yeah."

She was barely on the chair. With Dad still holding her shoulders, I dragged the chair a foot or so to the edge of the bed. Somehow we lifted her and got her almost to the center of the mattress. Her feet would have been hanging off the side if she hadn't kept her knees drawn up so tightly. She looked uncomfortable, but her smile came back.

"Is that okay, Mama?" I asked. I could go from irritation to acute concern with dizzying speed.

She just smiled. I put a pillow under her head and covered her with a clean sheet. She didn't move, didn't close her eyes, didn't watch me as I backed out of the room.

I found Dad at the kitchen table with his head in his hands.

"Uhhhhh," he muttered. No words, just misery.

I made us some tea and sat. The ubiquitous sound of news chattered in the background.

At last Dad turned from the TV to me. "She'll be all right now. She'll get up again after a while, and I'll get her pills into her with some water or more juice. Maybe she'll eat something."

I don't remember replying. I just stood and prepared to leave.

"You go on to work. We'll be fine. I sure do thank you for coming by and helping me." Dad's voice still had that sing-song tone. I heard despair which perhaps he didn't feel. Maybe that was only me.

"I'll come back by after work," I said. Time paused for a minute as I reached out to Dad with a look, long and direct.

Then I smiled. An honest smile. "We'll have snacks. Or something."

"Ok, baby." He mustered a chuckle. "Or something."

Dad accompanied me to the door as always. Stood on the porch as I got in my car. Waved as I backed out of the drive.

"I'll see you later!" I called, waving my arm out the window. And then for the hundredth, thousandth, millionth time, I imagined him turning his back to the world outside the door, returning to the table and his empty tea mug.

We had developed a habit, Dad and I, of never sharing negative things. We rejoiced together when the antidepressants helped, but we didn't cry to each other as we looked at Mom's poor hacked hair. We laughed and winked to each other as she delighted in the "new" roses for the third time in one afternoon, but I didn't ask him how he felt about having to scrub the carpet or the chair cushions again and again. I praised his patience and was endlessly cheerful in the most difficult times. But I never told him I was tired even if he wasn't, or that I wanted outside help for me and Mom even if he refused it for himself. I never invited him to speak of the pain, despair, and loneliness I knew he must be feeling, and I never mentioned my own.

Hiding those feelings from each other was a mistake. For myself, I can say that it left me utterly at the mercy of my imagination. I conjured up pictures of my parents' nonstop pain, pain that doubled or tripled each time I backed out of that driveway and left them alone. Maybe my imagination was correct, but I could have checked it out; I could have just asked Dad. Perhaps he would have confirmed my fears. But maybe he would have allayed them somehow.

Probably he would have lied to me, telling me he was fine, he was in control, everything was all right, I worried too much. But I wish I had invited him to share. I wish I'd been honest with him about how I felt and what I wanted and what I thought Mom needed, what all three of us needed. Maybe my honesty would have provoked his.

The sharing would have been as hard for me as for my father. I had installed myself in their lives like a handrail, to protect them from pain. Telling Dad about my frustration and fear would have caused him pain. But it would have been true, liberating, like a blast of winter cold through the door of a room where a fire has burned too hot for too long. Instead, Dad and I kept the doors to our pain closed and locked.

So, smiling and waving as usual, I left. When I got to work, I called Dad to see how things were going.

"She's okay," he assured me. "She's still resting."

Knowing he would call if there were any emergency, I focused on my work, thanking the Lord again for the blessing of this parttime job. It gave me structure. Sanity. Time in an environment where I had a measure of control.

I returned to my parents' house early that evening with a lighter heart. I was sure the morning's events were the worst we would see for this day and expected to find Mom sitting in her place at the table with Dad. I anticipated joining them there; maybe it would be a laid-back evening with some smiles and conversation before dinner.

I was wrong. Dad sat alone. Mom lay on the bed in the same position she had taken early in the morning.

Dad wasn't as concerned as I was. "She hasn't moved, hasn't had a thing to eat or drink all day, but she says she's fine."

Though the blinds were drawn, the late-day sun cut through the slats and made the bedroom overwarm. But somehow Mom looked cold beneath the pink and beige flowered sheet I'd put over her hours before. The heat had baked the smells of curtains, clothes, carpet, and mattress into a hardness that hit me again with each step I took into the room. From a million miles away, the TV news wandered in and drifted among the shafts of sunlight.

I bent over the bed with a smile and addressed Mom's blank gaze with the name she loved to hear me use. "How are you, one-that-borned-ed-me?" The flowery sheet remained unwrinkled, still creased with folds from the linen cabinet. Her pillow made a puffy halo around her head. I didn't expect her to answer me, but I waited just in case, searching in vain for any sign she had moved during the seven hours since I'd left her.

"Fine." Her answer, barely more than a breath, surprised me.

"Can you sit up and have a little something to drink?"

She smiled, said "No," and closed her eyes.

That was the end of the conversation. Nothing I said provoked any response beyond a tighter clenching of her eyelids.

When I returned to the breakfast room without her on my arm, Dad's face went blank with surprise. "You couldn't get her up?" His tone straddled anger and anxiety.

"No. We have to call the doctor, Daddy." I'm not sure when I decided that, but I was certain.

I turned down the volume of news of the world as I dialed the number. While I left a message with the doctor's after-hours service, I stared at Dad's head, cradled in his hands, shaking back and forth. I'd memorized all the geography of that globe.

"Oh, brother," he said. "What now?"

Next I called my sister. Expecting to have to leave a message, I was surprised to find her already home from work, then somehow remembered it was her wedding anniversary. I explained the situation to her and we decided I should call 9-1-1.

The call was simple. No long explanations required, just a brief statement of the facts and they were on their way. For a moment, I stood in the doorway of the bedroom and watched as Mom...what? Slept? I don't think so. I think she simply lay there and waited. As she had waited all day. I believe she would have died there, silent, waiting. For what? Or whom? She didn't know. On a different day she might have fought. Yelled. Something. But this day instinct abandoned her. So she waited. Help had always come before. I wonder if she remembered that as she lay there.

My sister arrived before the ambulance. She crawled up on the bed and put her face down at an angle to match Mom's. She spoke and Mom opened her eyes and smiled. I walked outside to move my car out of the drive, wondering if I should have crawled up on the bed, too.

The ambulance backed into the driveway; a fire truck parked at the curb. Although the evening was still young and bright, the emergency lights glared in circles around the neighborhood.

As the house exploded with activity, I realized I hadn't seen Dad in a while. Maybe he was trying to hide from the scene; I had already considered that option and, reluctantly, abandoned it.

Instead I shoved furniture aside to give the paramedics room to work. The bedroom filled with dark uniforms, sweaty foreheads, low voices, and more heat. Two paramedics leaned over the bed where Mom still lay, eyes open, with my sister right beside her. I listened from the hallway, looking up at the ceiling where an attic fan used to be.

On stifling afternoons in my teenage years, I used to bring my pillow and a book and lie on the floor under the soft breeze from the fan. Often I fell asleep, but never for long; Mom would see me there and tell me to get up. The fan was gone now, replaced by an attic stairway and central air-conditioning.

From my place in the hall, I answered questions coming from the bedroom: the doctor's name, how long Mom had been in bed, what she'd had to eat and drink. I heard the medics ask Mom if she wanted to go to the hospital. My sister answered that the doctor had already told us to bring her there. Actually, we hadn't heard back from the doctor yet, but I saw no reason to clear up this minor miscommunication. Mom needed to go; clearly an ambulance would be necessary; the paramedics were ready to take her.

The next challenge became finding a way to move Mom from her awkward spot in the middle of the bed. She didn't seem willing or able to move herself and the paramedics were reluctant to disturb her apparently pain-free position. They solved the problem by gently lifting the four sides of the sheet beneath her and lowering her to the gurney. Dad observed the maneuver from the corner where he'd been standing all this time.

The ambulance drove down the neighborhood street with lights on, but no siren. My sister and Dad and I followed in the car, mystified. A stroke? Or maybe Mom had hit her head when she fell?

Predictably, Dad fumed. He was always angry when Mom was hurt, the level of his fury in direct proportion to his perception of the seriousness of her injury. On my middle son's fourth birthday, an icy January morning twenty years before, Mom fell on the steps of my back porch and cut her head. Dad was furious with both her and me for hours. Days. But this time he must have been confused about where to point his ire. He sighed and fidgeted but remained silent.

The short distance to the hospital took us down roads Mom used to drive almost daily. Past the McDonald's where she bought french fries for my boys, telling them she couldn't control her car—it made the turn in to McDonald's all by itself! My youngest believed with wide eyes and a wider smile. The oldest, proud to be in on the story, grinned and winked at me. And the middle son kept to his usual place—between them—not sure he believed, but not sure Gramma was entirely in control. There was wisdom in his doubting.

Just a little past the drive-through entrance, we turned to the left and entered the hospital grounds. One more quick turn and we arrived at the emergency entrance, where the silent blink of the ambulance lights beat against the wall of the hospital. I willed the lights to stop, give me time to think, but they throbbed on as we parked. Red and blue, bright and dark, they took their turns at the wall while paramedics took Mom on the gurney through a staff-only door.

The ambulance driver directed us to a sidewalk that led to the main door of the emergency room. Smokers were clustered close to the entrance. They moved aside and looked down as Dad passed them, with Sis and me following right behind.

After completing the admission papers, we were allowed to join Mom in an examining room. I feared an interminable wait for a physician, but at least we had the privacy of a room. I couldn't imagine Mom tolerating the crowded waiting room for any length of time. Full of sick people, it teemed with activity: people coming in, moving through, going out. Parents scolding, or not scolding, their children. Tears, laughter, cell phone conversations, the never-ending blare of a television. Mom would have hated it. Or maybe she would have loved it. Either way, she would have had lots to say to everyone: growling and scowling at the children, endless questions and commands for us.

By contrast, silence dominated our wait in the cold exam room. Down the hall and outside the double doors, our husbands and children gathered, in person or on the phone. But in here we were only four again, the family pared down to the nucleus of my childhood. Mom lying silent but restless. Dad sighing and pacing, jingling the change in his pockets. My sister and I sitting, one of us in the room's lone chair and the other on a round revolving stool. I bounced my legs on the balls of my feet. Sis, on the stool, swiveled back and forth in quick quarter-turns.

Occasionally our eyes met. If Dad had his back to us, we'd shake our heads or lift our eyebrows, or both, then close our eyes for a second or two, with some dragging our fingers through our hair thrown in for good measure. It was a silent conversation, not unlike the whispered ones we'd engaged in growing up, the two of us on the outside looking in at the private room of my parents' marriage. We were of it but never in it, a reality imposed on us very early in our lives. So we forged our own unit, Sis and I, functioning with a closeness and loyalty that rivaled my parents' union. Later our own marriages and families stretched our tight bond almost to breaking, but as we sat shivering in the chill of the room and the circumstance, the comfort of the old ties rushed back to warm me. To warm us both, I think.

The young doctor who examined my mother was a surprise. A gift. A miracle. He still stands out among the many doctors I have met in emergency rooms before and since. His bedside manner easily accommodated my mother's silence. Maybe his training as a hospital generalist had included a special unit on dealing with patients with dementia. Maybe he simply had a way with elderly patients. No matter what, he was a miracle. Gentle, genial, unflappable. He ordered tests and scans, and asked questions Mom pretended not to hear. We did our best to answer on her behalf.

Hours passed. In the cold ivory room, small events drew our immediate and focused attention: a faraway siren, the delivery of another blanket for my mother, Dad's grin after his "theft" of a vacant chair from the hall outside, my sister's discovery of a coffee machine, a muffled laugh from an adjoining room. Sometime close to midnight, the doctor took Sis, Dad, and me out into the hall. He finally had a diagnosis: broken hip.

A broken hip? Astounding. The morning seemed days ago. Mom had lain all day, all evening, and now well into the night...with a broken hip. She had sat upright for a few minutes, had even stood, with our support, for ten seconds or so. She had not complained of the slightest pain, even when Dad and I moved her to the bed.

The doctor, who looked at us with eyes still bright and alert at this late, or early, hour, whose tone still showed interest and care, continued to talk while my thoughts stayed riveted on his first words. I tuned back in as he explained that Mom's injury was "not good, not good at all."

"Can't it be fixed?" Dad asked.

"Yes, with surgery," the doctor replied. But Mom's chances of successful rehabilitation after the surgery were very slim, he explained. And certainly the surgery itself would not be easy on her. Though surprisingly healthy for her age, she *was* eighty-two, and frail. And Alzheimer's posed a major complication to her recovery and rehabilitation.

The alternative to repairing her hip? Keep her comfortable. In bed. She would be bedridden for the rest of her life.

Dad had fought Mom's monsters for so long as they ripped away pieces of her mind, her life. Each piece of her that vanished carried a piece of his heart with it. How, then, could he still have enough heart left to feel the pain I read now on his face?

"Oh, no," he said, in a tone that asked how the doctor could even suggest such a thing. "No. We can't leave her like that. No."

I stood speechless in the face of his devastation. I couldn't muster a word of encouragement or advice. Not even a question.

My sister, on the other hand, an expert in the field of medical records, knew what to ask. She questioned the doctor in a language I scarcely heard and didn't understand. "Well, Daddy," she finally said, "we might have to consider—"

"No," Dad interrupted her. "We can't leave her this way."

The doctor repeated questions he had asked earlier: Could Mom walk? Did she get any exercise?

"Oh, yes! She walks everywhere!" Dad replied. "She can walk fine!"

Sis and I exchanged a look. *"Can."* Ability was one thing. Willingness was something else entirely. We were challenged to achieve Mom's cooperation on a good day. What would it take to gain it after this?

The doctor explained that not being able to sit up in bed after the surgery and during rehabilitation would bring a whole new set of threats to Mom's health. Dad assured him that Mom could and would sit up for as long as necessary.

And so Dad and the doctor made the final decision. Since Mom had been ambulatory prior to this accident, there was "sufficient justification," the doctor said, for replacing the hip joint and attempting rehab. He would put Mom in traction for a day or two to stabilize the hip before surgery.

The joy I saw in Dad's blue eyes could have lit the hallway. "Good!" he boomed. Then, more quietly, "Good! I know she can do it!"

By the time Mom was admitted and settled into a room, the clock had slid around to no-man's-land. The dark before the dawn. The wee hours of a new day.

Time to get Dad home.

Our husbands and families had left after the diagnosis, so just the three of us made the long walk back through the now-empty emergency room, through the quiet ambulance pavilion, and out to the almost-deserted parking lot. None of us had eaten; no one had an appetite now. We drove straight to my parents' house and made plans to meet at the hospital in a few hours.

Dad's parting words gave no indication of the bone-deep fatigue and anxiety he had to be feeling. "She can do it," he repeated. "I know she can do it. We can't leave her like that. We have to try."

He was right, of course. We had to try.

NOTES

> Most important to note, **Dad and I should have called Mom's doctor that morning before trying to lift her.** The doctor would surely have told us to call the paramedics and let them check her out. We could have aggravated Mom's injury by lifting her, asking her to try to stand, letting her sit down, then putting her on the bed. The difficult fact is we didn't know what had happened, only that she couldn't or wouldn't stand. The possibility of a broken

bone never entered our minds. In hindsight, we reminded ourselves: calling the professionals is *always* the best course. A person with Alzheimer's has limited understanding and limited speech, at best. So in a case of possible injury, there's almost always doubt. **When in doubt, call the professionals.**

➤ Dad and I still felt anger at some of Mom's actions, even when we were certain she couldn't control them. Our anger was like a reflex, an immediate reaction to difficult behaviors and seemingly impossible situations. Don't be surprised if you feel the same kind of anger or doubt. We can't control what we feel, but we can control what we do. And what we must do is always assume it's the disease that's acting, not our loved ones.

➤ I wish I had been more honest about my feelings. I kept all my pain, anger, fatigue, guilt, doubt, and despair inside. I could have talked about them to the rest of my family, my friends, or my support group. I could have invited Dad to share his feelings with me. Instead I tried to appear upbeat all the time. It wasn't the truth. I pray you will say what you're feeling. Say what's true. It really does set us free.

➤ As your loved one's health deteriorates, you will likely come up against decisions you feel you cannot make. When I was in that position, I prayed. And then, having prayed, I trusted the doctor. Perhaps surgery wasn't the best choice for my mother. But it was the best decision we could make for her at that time. And God was able to make it right, to make it yield the best results for my mother. He will do the same for you.

Fighting

Do not be afraid of them; the Lord your
God himself will fight for you.
—DEUTERONOMY 3:22, NIV

Early morning light shone into the room in the northeast corner of the second floor. It barely penetrated the three feet or so of beige linoleum between the window and the hospital bed. Metal bars, sprouting up from the bed frame, held square gray slabs in careful balance with the weight of Mom's left leg. The bed itself was a fortress of cotton-white pillows, carefully arranged to protect and immobilize Mom's leg and the broken hip joint that connected it to the rest of her body. She was asleep.

I stood just inside the doorway. Now that I'd located Mom's room, Dad took the lead. He pushed past me, but slowed his steps as he walked farther in, between a sink and mirror on the right and a blank wall on the left. Turning away from the window's hazy view, he faced the tight formation of IV poles and lines surrounding the head of the bed. A rolling table stood nearby, covered with cups, towels, and breathing contraptions.

Dad ran his fingertips over the metal scaffold and blue slings of the traction assembly, then looked at Mom's closed eyes and smiled. "Oh, she's sleeping just fine." Her small form was arranged among the pillows, her hands lying atop unwrinkled white sheets. Dad bent, kissed the air above her face, backed away from the bed, and turned to where I still stood in the doorway. "Let's get some breakfast while she's sleeping!"

Jingling the change in his pockets and backing toward the door, Dad seemed anxious to leave. But we needed—well, I needed—to know Mom's status before we did anything or went anywhere. Maybe Dad feared the night had been difficult and he didn't want to know. Or maybe his perennial hopefulness made him certain all had gone well.

That's what I wanted: certainty. Certainty that this peaceful scene would last. Mom here in this strange place, among strangers, contained in a hospital bed and sleeping—the miracle of it amazed me. I was immeasurably grateful that she appeared to be in no distress, either physical or mental. Still, how long would it last? I wanted to be prepared for what the day ahead might bring.

The nurse's arrival at just that moment kept me from having to persuade Dad to wait. I expected to see tension in her eyes or hear frustration in her voice, but those were, apparently, my emotions. Despite having cared for Mom during the dark hours of the night and early morning, the nurse smiled as Dad and I introduced ourselves.

In my memory, her voice remains a soft blanket of competence and care. "Mrs. Bailey has been just fine," she assured my father. "I understand she had a long hard day yesterday and then a long evening in the ER, so she's just worn out. She'll probably sleep until early afternoon, at least."

The nurse explained the traction assembly and went over Mom's medications. She applauded Dad's decision to get some breakfast, noting that the surgeon would be in later in the day to talk to us.

I could tell Dad's broken heart was on the mend. Walking with square shoulders toward the elevator, "Forgot to shave this morning, baby!" he announced to me and to the nurses, doctors, and visitors in the hallway and the patients in the rooms who had not had the forethought to close their doors before LJ Bailey came to visit his wife. "I'm sorry! I'll shave for sure tomorrow!"

I imagined he was already seeing Mom sitting across the table from him, perhaps dipping potato chips into her tepid tea, but hip healed and working fine. Now he rubbed his stubbly chin while we waited for the elevator. On the ride down he invited everyone aboard to join us for breakfast.

In spite of Dad's cheer, I felt a pang of guilt with each step we walked toward the cafeteria. Not for leaving Mom in a foreign environment in the care of people she wouldn't recognize, but for leaving those strangers at the mercy of the monster disease that had stolen Mom's life. I thought they couldn't possibly know what they were in for when she awakened. They wouldn't be able to handle her without me or my father there. Having surrendered for so long to Dad's insistence that we needed no help, I had finally convinced myself no outside help was possible. I anticipated the situation here would be the same as at home: Dad and I on Alzheimer's duty. While the doctors and hospital staff treated my mother's broken hip, we would deal with the monster.

We.

I.

Dad found breakfast in the hospital cafeteria so delicious and so reasonably priced, he decided the workers in nearby businesses should come to the hospital to eat lunch. "People living around here should consider it a restaurant!" he declared. "I would, if your mother and I lived closer."

I agreed with him, as I always did.

When we returned to the second floor after breakfast, I listened closely. I heard televisions and bedside conversations and the breathing of machinery, but I didn't hear what I expected: I didn't hear my mother's voice, hoarse with rage. Looking down the length of the hall, I saw white coats and multicolored uniforms moving in and out of rooms, but no frantic activity around the room in the northeast corner. Dad exhaled through pursed lips as we walked the last few yards. I followed him into the room.

Mom slept on. Her face the color of sandy soil and cigarette ash against the extreme white of the pillowcase, her hair lying lifeless against her scalp, her lips open but sagging onto poor naked gums, she slept.

This time my father kissed her cheek. "How doin', honey?" he murmured into her face.

She opened her eyes and smiled. One finger fluttered for a second on the sheet, a move approximating the tapping of a cigarette against an ashtray.

"Fine, Daddy."

No questions. No outrage. No fear. Just "fine." I could see it. She was fine.

The nurse came in, a cup of ice chips in her hand. "Oh, we've had a nice conversation."

Mom's face brightened as at the appearance of a long lost friend. My face probably looked the same as I smiled in the nurse's direction.

Moods and hours would pass. Light would gather and grow dim. But for this moment, the monster had surrendered to a force I hadn't had to muster, and I rejoiced in the miracle. I surrendered to the unfamiliar but wholly pleasant feeling of relief and let the professional army take over.

The surgeon was a youngish doctor who appeared to house enormous energy and knowledge in his compact frame. As he addressed my father, the swift gallop of his speech slowed to a moderate walk. At first he spoke with his hands thrust deep in the starched pockets of his white coat, but as he described the surgery, he began gesturing. Dad interrupted occasionally with questions that revealed his interest in every detail of the mechanics of hip joint repair. At that point, the doctor grabbed a blue marker from the tray below the message board and drew with dark, solid strokes. Two things became clear during their animated conversation: Dad was fascinated with the engineering of the new joint and the doctor was surprised and impressed by his questions. I watched them, the young surgeon and the veteran aeronautical engineer, with pleasure and pride for Dad's eighty-five-year-old intellect that refused to stop learning.

Mom drifted off to sleep again and the surgery was scheduled for the next afternoon.

By early evening, Mom was awake and showing signs of wear. Far past being able to ask where she was, she simply repeated again and again: "I want to go home." Her hands wandered across the bedcovers. Her legs, held in the fortress of bars and pillows, gave a twitch now and then that caused her to look in their direction. "Water?" I offered periodically. "Ice?" Dad asked. A loud "Leave me be!" was Mom's only answer, if she answered us at all. So we did.

My sister had joined us by now and the three of us talked of weather and world events and parking spaces in the hospital lot. Sometimes we could coax a smile out of our patient with stories about Charley-Dog, waiting like a good boy at home, peeing on the hem of the beige rocking chair and sleeping on Mom's sofa. Of course, we didn't actually mention the peeing. Mom couldn't make sense of most of our words and wouldn't have believed it of the angelic Charley anyway. What she did understand, I think, was Charley's name and the smile in our voices as we said it.

As medical personnel came and went, I noted that, as far as the staff was concerned, Dad's decision for surgery had moved Mom from the category of "patient with Alzheimer's," not to "patient with Alzheimer's and a broken hip," but simply "patient with a broken hip." This disease had dominated our lives for so long, I expected it to be the first thought on the mind of these professional caregivers as well. I waited for them to ask about her mental capabilities, her mood changes, what they should anticipate. But they just saw her as someone to be cared for, like the man down the hall with a knee replacement or the woman next door scheduled to have her gallbladder removed. Surely, there had to be a note on her chart about Alzheimer's, but at this point it seemed to have no greater implications than a note about her cholesterol or her persistent eye infection.

Meanwhile, I marveled at Mom's reaction to the nurses' care. She cooperated completely, with blood draws and temperature checks, even the wipe-down that passed for a bath and left her cleaner than she'd been in a month. Would she have tolerated this at home? So much body contact and social interaction? Perhaps, but only on rare occasions. For some time before Mom fell, I'd been convinced that a professional caregiver would be more effective with her in the long term than Dad or I. Now, as I watched these nurses care for her, I remembered Montsie.

Montsie was an aide I had persuaded Dad to hire. Actually, I hired her and told Dad she was coming. She worked with us at my parents' home for two brief afternoons.

The first day, Mom was uncooperative, but not out of control. She would do better, Montsie advised us, if Dad and I left for a while. "Take a break!" she told us. "That's why I'm here, so you can get a break. Go out and see something new, do something different. I can do my job. We'll be fine together, better than if you're here."

I knew leaving Mom alone with Montsie would be a hard sell, but I thought I could persuade Dad to at least go for a cup of coffee and a piece of pie. He usually found the prospect of cherry pie well-nigh irresistible. But no. He would go no farther away than the patio in back of the house. He sat out there 'til Montsie left.

At the end of the second day of Montsie's three-days-a-week assignment with us, Dad told her not to come back. He insisted Mom "just couldn't tolerate" anyone but him or me. So the capable Montsie never had a chance. Dad didn't want her there and I didn't assert myself to make him do what I knew would be better for all of us.

Now, here in the hospital, none of us had a choice. The nurses cared for Mom well and she gave them very little trouble. I wondered again what improvements could have been accomplished in each of our lives if Montsie had been given the opportunity to do her job.

By the next day, the day of the surgery, Mom had virtually stopped reacting. I imagined confusion and discomfort overwhelmed her. Or perhaps this accident had happened at the precise moment when Alzheimer's was poised to carry her even further away from us. Maybe her fall and the break resulted from a shift in the disease. But regardless of the cause of her fall, I believe the physical trauma and the onslaught of sensory experiences that barraged her body and mind after she broke her hip accelerated her decline into a deeper stage of the disease.

Early on the day of the surgery, Mom was given pre-surgery medication, intended in part to relax her, though she'd been virtually silent for the last twelve hours. At the appointed time, two surgical technicians, wearing blue scrubs, stethoscopes, and tennis shoes, strode with kind efficiency into the room. They made quick work of the IV lines and oxygen tubes, then pushed the big, barred bed past me and my sister. Dad stood closer to the door, by the sink where unused toothpaste lay beside unopened mouthwash. The march to surgery paused while he kissed Mom's forehead. "See you later, honey. I sure do love you." After waiting a few seconds for a response Mom never gave, the aides pushed the bed into the hallway. By the time the door clicked shut, Dad had moved to the window, where he watched a helicopter with a red cross on its side slowly circle the hospital.

"Oh, look at that. Somebody must be in really bad shape. I feel sorry for that family." He shook his head and sighed. "We're so lucky."

NOTES

- Dad expected Mom to reject any kind of care from someone other than him or me. Instead, she accepted, usually without question, whatever the hospital staff did for her or to her.
- If your loved one is hospitalized, be prepared for your role to change. I had to monitor myself—actually *remind* myself to keep out of the way. Several times I folded my hands behind my back to slow the urge to help. I thanked the Lord for the nurses' competence and stepped away from the bed.
- I expected Mom's behavior would irritate the hospital staff. I feared Alzheimer's would interfere with their schedules and complicate their routines. But even when Mom was uncooperative, things went smoothly. For the first time, I could see firsthand the benefits of bringing professionals in to take charge of some aspects of Mom's care.
- If you do bring helpers into your home, give them time— and space—to do their jobs. Although a professional caregiver can make caring for your loved one easier in the long run, the benefits may not be immediately apparent. At first, the change may cause added tension, as change of any kind often does. You may find yourself nervous, and your loved one may be restless, even angry. But you may be confident that professional caregivers anticipate such reactions. They are trained to work through the initial uncertainty of new clients. Give them time to make the process work for your loved one and for you.

➤ Whether they are professionals or volunteers, it's wise to have supplies ready for helpers to use in your home. Disposable gloves, cleaning supplies, and a description of a typical day's routine will help make the first days go more smoothly. Depending on your loved one's needs and wants, you could leave the caregiver with photo albums, familiar music, even the ingredients for a favorite meal.

➤ When a caregiver is there to help your loved one, you don't have to leave your house, or even leave the room. Especially in the beginning, you will almost certainly want to observe the interaction between helper and client. But be aware, many caregivers say it's easier for them to get to know the client in a one-on-one setting.

➤ The caregiver will come to know your loved one well, and your loved one will likely come to feel as safe with the caregiver as with you. In addition, you will benefit from taking a break. Getting out of the house, being with friends, enjoying exercise and the stimulation of friends and activity, even simply retiring to another room to read, watch television, or talk on the phone can refresh you and allow you to return to caregiving with new energy.

Steps

The Lord makes firm the steps of the one who delights in him; though he
may stumble, he will not fall, for the Lord upholds him with his hand.
—PSALM 37:23–24, NIV

Mom's hip was replaced with titanium, strong enough, Dad said, to last forever. After the surgery, she slept through the evening and then all night.

The next morning, either still asleep or only on the edge of consciousness, Mom got busy. Her hands held the loose end of the bed sheet while her fingers folded the hem into careful pleats. How many times had I watched Mom sitting at her sewing machine, pinning pleats in place, or darts, or interfacing, or lining. Having no pins here for the hospital sheet made things very convenient—as her fingers moved across the fabric, the pleats formed, then fell away, and when her hands went back to the beginning, they found more work to do. Pleat, move on, go back. Pleat, move on, go back.

The traction apparatus had disappeared. Now specially shaped foam pillows hugged Mom's legs and torso to keep the new hip in place. They did their job at first, but her habit of crossing her legs at the knees kicked in about twenty-four hours after the surgery. At home, moving her legs, crossing and uncrossing them in rapid, jerky movements, was a way Mom reacted to stress. Beneath the covers, her legs tried to do the same here, making us all wince, making my father frantic.

"Baby, you can't *do* that! It looks like the pain would *kill* you!"

The nurse gave us strict instructions more than once: "Well, Mrs. Bailey, you've got these pillows knocked everywhere again. Y'all really need to try and keep her legs right where I put them so that hip heals right."

So my sister took over the discipline department. "Now Mama, you just can't do that," she would state in my mother's own stern tone. "You'll never get out of here if that hip doesn't work correctly."

But neither pain, nor pleading, nor inherited unquestioned authority could keep those legs from crossing. Finally, soft, velcro-fastened straps held them in place...at which point the level of tension in the room in the northeast corner escalated quickly.

Mom, of course, understood nothing of the hip's need to heal. Awake, alert, and angry at being restrained, she managed, to some extent at least, to defeat the straps. She simply moved her upper body instead of her legs. We did what we could, short of using full-body restraints, to keep her positioned more or less correctly more or less of the time.

Mom got little rest. We got none.

On the morning of the third day after surgery, after Dad and I had our usual delicious and economical breakfast, we returned to find Mom sitting on the side of the bed. A wide, woven-cloth belt hung loosely around her waist. One of two physical therapists held onto the belt with a firm grasp, his eyes fixed on my mother's face smiling up at him like a child's.

The two young men, both in pressed khaki pants and polo shirts, were coaxing and coaching. "A little this way...oh, wait now, you're leaning over again...remember what we said? Therrrrre you go...great! That's great!" They applauded what I imagined had to be a mammoth effort on Mom's part.

Dad and I stood in the doorway hoping not to be seen, both of us amazed at the scene before us: Mom not only sitting up, but cooperating, smiling.

Next, the therapists positioned themselves in mirrored stances, one on either side of Mom, each grasping one side of the woven belt. With a slow but steady movement, like the opening of a flower, she stood.

"Yay!" My father clapped and cheered. "You did it, baby! Look at that! You did it! You stood right up!"

Mom turned her head slowly as if waking from sleep. Still smiling, she nodded and leaned to the side like the Tower of Pisa.

"Whoa!" the dark-haired therapist said in a tone modulated by what had to be extreme self-control. Feet planted, one of their arms under each of hers, the two of them lowered her to the bed and caught her as she fell limp across its width. I expected at least a grimace of pain while they lifted and moved her and repositioned the pillows and the straps, but her face betrayed nothing. She closed her eyes and the therapists beckoned us to follow as they left the room.

His loud enthusiasm not the least bit modulated in the quiet hallway, Dad leaned forward and bent his knees slightly as if that would accentuate his words: "You guys are *great!* Wasn't that fine? She even stood up! I was so worried—I thought she might not walk again. You guys are the best!"

By now he was grabbing their hands, shaking first one, then the other. The "guys" were trying to talk but hadn't been able to yet. The dark-haired one tried again. Now I could see the name on the badge attached to his shirt: Curtis.

"Yes, Mr. Bailey," Curtis said, "she did really well. We weren't too sure at first; we couldn't get her to open her eyes for us yesterday."

"You guys were here yesterday? Well, where was I? Why weren't we here?" Dad's eyes shot my direction and I felt accused.

As I tried to remember some vestige of the day before, Curtis rescued me. "The nurse told us you all had gone to dinner just before we got here. We were going to introduce ourselves but she said you'd just left. Anyway, obviously we didn't get anything done yesterday, but she did fine today." He went on to explain that someone else would be in later in the day to repeat the exercises.

"It's important for her to be able to do the rehab," his partner added.

"Oh, she can do it!" Dad replied, his voice colored not with hope but with absolute conviction. "She can do it."

I thought I saw more hope than certainty in Curtis's face as he waved and headed for the nurses' station. But I was fresh from witnessing for myself Mom's cooperation and her physical strength. I didn't know which surprised me more, which was the greater miracle. I prayed with gratitude for each, for both, and for Dad's newly squared shoulders and lighter step.

That evening, as the new therapist stood in the doorway introducing herself to Dad, Mom suddenly "fell asleep." The slim young woman had dark hair wrapped in a bun on top of her head and a wide woven belt hanging loose across her shoulders. Undeterred, she began talking to Mom the moment she crossed the threshold. Her warm voice matched her slow stride.

"Hi, Mrs. Bailey! I'm Sarah. I'm going to help you get up for a little while." By this time, she was leaning slightly over the bed. "Mrs. Bai-ley…".

Mom opened her eyes for a second, then slammed them shut again.

"Mrs. Bailey? This won't take long. Just a little exercise. To make you strong again." Sarah was stroking Mom's hand as she talked. "They told me you did really well this morning! I'm excited to see you try again. Can you open your eyes?"

"C'mon, baby!" Dad leaned over from the other side of the bed. "Let me see you do it again!"

No response. No movement.

"Marie! Come on, baby." Dad bent very close to Mom's face and spoke in a loud whisper. "You need to do this, baby. So you can get out of here and come home with me and Charley-Dog."

Still no response.

"Okay, Mrs. Bailey." Sarah made her voice all disappointment. "I guess I'll leave now. Are you sure you don't want to wake up and move around a little?"

With her eyes still tightly closed, Mom pulled her left hand from beneath Sarah's hovering touch. I sighed but had to smile at the sight of my mother's arm stretched awkwardly across the top of the blue blanket, angling sharply away from Sarah's voice and fingers. I was familiar from childhood with my mother's ability to speak without words. She had spoken. Sarah left.

A faint shade of the summer sunset somehow rounded the brick corners of the hospital, then traveled with quick steps across the black-graveled roof, clambered silently through the half-open blinds, and lay down on the floor of the room in the northeast corner. We sat in it, Dad and I, quiet as the light.

The morning after Sarah's aborted therapy visit, we arrived extra early, made quick work of breakfast, and hurried back to Mom's room, where Dad, a firm believer in schedules, intended to wait for Curtis and his partner. I knew, however, that schedules in a hospital are rigid as bed rails when it comes to taking vital signs and dispensing medications. Meal deliveries and operating rooms function within predictable boundaries, like the acceptable ranges of blood pressure and body temperature. But on-time visits from therapists and social workers are only as reliable as a noncommittal prognosis. And seeing the patient's doctor is like waiting up for Santa Claus: you assume he or she will be there within a rough twelve-hour time span. You have to believe. You just believe.

Dad believed the therapists would arrive at the same time as the day before. Instead, we almost missed them. They were leaving Mom's room when we returned from breakfast. And it was not Curtis and his partner, but two new faces. Before they could speak, Dad's anxiety and frustration burst over them.

"*Oh no!* I knew we'd miss you guys! How long have you been here? You weren't anywhere around when we left and we've only been gone—what, Katrinka?—fifteen minutes? You're leaving? How did she do?"

"I think it was closer to half an hour," I interposed, anxious to protect these strangers from my father's anger. As usual, I found myself in the middle, stretched thin, trying to close the gap between the frustration and fear behind Dad's loud outbursts and the usually detached professionalism of these people formally charged with my mother's care. I feared the scene Dad could create in this quiet hallway with so many sick people behind so many doors. I was afraid these two therapists, whose success with Mom was so important, would give up on this difficult family and just walk away.

They didn't.

The brightest light in the galaxy of blessings that shone on us during my mother's hospitalization was the patience of the caregivers we encountered. Through the gathering darkness of Mom's fear and pain and confusion, their care and understanding and compassion shone through like starlight.

"I'm Robert. You must be Mr. Bailey." A man about Dad's height with blue eyes looking out from wire-rimmed glasses held out his hand and continued talking. "Mrs. Bailey did fine this morning. She's pretty tired, and I think she's in some pain, but she did her best."

"Oh, that's fine!" Relief filled Dad's quiet words, spoken as he peered through the doorway toward the bed.

Robert stepped closer and leaned to the side, putting his face squarely into Dad's line of sight.

"Mr. Bailey," he said, "rehab is very hard for Alzheimer's patients."

Robert's assistant, silent and anonymous, backed away from the conversation, then turned and walked down the hall. I didn't want to watch my father's reaction to what Robert was saying, so I kept my eyes focused on the assistant's back, shrinking smaller and smaller as he walked away.

"Rehab is hard for anyone who's broken a hip," Robert continued, "but it's especially difficult for Alzheimer's patients. They have to be able to remember how to move, like which leg to move first, and how it should feel, how to balance before they step or sit down. They have to be able to do the exercises a couple of hours a day, every single day. That's a lot; it takes endurance."

"Mm-hmm. I see." Dad stared at the floor. "So. You're saying she can't do it."

"I'm saying it's hard for her. When she tries, it's very hard. And sometimes she doesn't even feel like trying."

"Mm-hmm. I see." Head still down, Dad was trying to concede defeat. But then he looked straight into Robert's wire-rimmed glasses. "Do you think she can do it?"

And then Robert blinked. "I'll talk to the doctor," he said, holding out his hand to Dad. "We're going to talk about the best way...the best way to help Mrs. Bailey. Okay?" With one hand grasping Dad's, Robert put the other on Dad's shoulder and bent far down to meet the older pair of blue eyes which were turned again to the floor.

"All right!" Dad looked up with a forced smile. "You betcha! Thanks a million, Robert."

The familiar tone of my father's pain stabbed me. I knew that fake smile and the badly acted can-do attitude. They made my heart sink like a waterlogged coat, dragging me down in waters the depth of which I, like my father, had up to now refused to acknowledge.

There was no therapy visit that evening. And we stayed late, but the doctor visited sometime after we left. The day must have been even longer for him than it was for us.

NOTES

> The frustration of missing the doctor's or therapists' daily visits could have been avoided if I had asked the nurses to call my cell phone when the doctor was on the floor. Such an obvious solution, using a cell phone to communicate within the walls of the hospital, but it didn't occur to me at the time. By the way, this is the kind of suggestion you would likely hear at a support group meeting.

> I wasn't prepared for the obstacles Alzheimer's would put in the way of Mom's recovery. Physical endurance and the ability to understand instructions, remember them, and cooperate with therapists are essential elements for successful physical rehabilitation. Moreover, in the case of almost any illness or injury, the patient's overall strength, conditioning, and attitude are critically important to recovery and recuperation. A person with Alzheimer's often has little strength, mental or physical, to contribute to the healing.

> Remember that serious illness or injury usually doesn't give a warning. You may want to talk to your physician and your support group about the health problems that can hasten the decline of someone with Alzheimer's. That knowledge will help you make more informed decisions if you have to face one of those problems.

Looking for the Exit

They will come with weeping; they will pray as I bring them back.
I will lead them beside streams of water on a level path where
they will not stumble....I will turn their mourning into gladness;
I will give them comfort and joy instead of sorrow.
—JEREMIAH 31:9, 13, NIV

T he next morning, Dad, Sis, and I had breakfast at the hospital again. But it wasn't the same. The smell of soapy dishcloths and burned bacon overpowered the aroma of hot coffee that usually greeted us. Humidity, excessive on that day even by Texas standards, had oozed its way in at the hospital entrance with each spin of the revolving doors. And here in the cafeteria it sank, fetid with grease and steam, onto every surface: blue tabletops, brown trays, beige floors.

We sat in our regular spot, but in silence. Apparently we weren't the only diners with spirits weighed down; in this normally cheerful room, conversation was sparse, laughter nonexistent. At our table, though no one said it, I knew we were mourning the death of hope. I looked around at the other people eating and drinking, heads down, quiet, and I wondered what else had died.

When we reached the northeast corner of the second floor, Mom lay with her eyes closed, her fingers deftly pleating the sheet again. At our greeting, she glanced up with a pleasant look. Not smiling, but pleasant. She was wearing her dentures today. Without them, she had been an extreme caricature of wrinkled and demented old age. With them, stained and ill-fitting as they were, she was more my mother.

Sis bent and kissed her forehead. "Well, how are you this morning?" she asked.

The pleating stopped. "Just fine," Mom breathed.

Again I was stung by the glow that seemed to come over her face when Sis visited. My sister could almost always draw Mom out of whatever fog she was in. Her confusion or anger or oblivion would lift for a bit and a look of recognition, a timeless knowing, would warm her features and her eyes.

My sister's was a newer face, I told myself. While Dad and I were as ubiquitous as the pills Mom didn't want to take, the clothes she didn't want to change, the food she didn't want to eat, Sis was still "company," which meant she merited the greatly improved mood and manners reserved for visitors. And even as the company manners faded with the progression of the disease, Sis retained her charm.

Because, of course, she wasn't just a newer face. She had that other allure—she would always be the firstborn. The first magic my parents had made from their love. I knew this. I believed it and understood it. I was even grateful for it, that look of recognition and pleasure on Mom's face. But it stung.

I was standing nearest the door when the social worker walked in.

"Julie," she introduced herself and shook my hand. Young, dressed in a short black skirt and a silky blouse, with her hospital ID hanging from a black cord around her neck, she had a lovely smile and warm brown eyes. I introduced Dad, Sis, and, lastly, Mom, whose eyes were now tightly closed.

Julie pulled a wooden folding chair toward the window side of the room, where Dad sat on its twin. She faced him, put her elbows on her knees, and ignored the clipboard in her lap. I recognized the top sheet on the clipboard; it was a form Sis and I had filled out in the earliest hours of the day Mom was admitted to the hospital.

The form asked questions about what Mom's living arrangements had been before this hospitalization. Did she live at home? Alone? With someone? A spouse? Did she need help? Eating? Bathing? Dressing? Did she have help? It asked about her religious preference and her mental status. Then it asked what kind of help she would need when she was discharged from the hospital. How much help, it asked. We had left those last questions unanswered.

But Julie ignored the form. She leaned toward my father, put one of her hands on his arm, and asked, "How are you doing, Mr. Bailey?"

"Doing fine, Judy. I'm doing just fine." He said it quietly, as though resigned to the necessity of being fine, in spite of the profound uncertainty of his life with my mother. Of his life.

Julie didn't correct him when he got her name wrong. I loved her for that and for meeting his gaze and for seeing that most of the real suffering in this room was his.

"Mr. Bailey, I think Mrs. Bailey will be released from the hospital tomorrow. She'll need to go to a nursing facility—you and she live alone, right?"

He lowered his eyes. The slightest of pauses marked his taking in the words that ended his fantasy of life going back to normal.

"Well, there's Charley-Dog," he said with a grim chuckle.

His hands rested in his lap, palm to palm, as though he was praying. But his fingers were spread, and he drummed them together, pinkie to pinkie, ring to ring, middle to middle, and index to index. Again and again, thumbs unmoving.

"Yes. We live alone. I've been taking care of Marie. Still can!" With these last two words, Dad lifted his head to look up at her, his eyebrows raised in a question, with a small smile which Julie returned in kind.

"I wish you could, Mr. Bailey, but she's going to need too much. Not skilled nursing, but lots of care. More than you can give."

"Not skilled nursing?" Sis seemed familiar with the term and jumped on it. "Rehab?"

"Rehab isn't really an option for Mrs. Bailey." Julie looked to my sister, then turned back to Dad. "For rehab, she needs to be able to remember, Mr. Bailey. Do the same things over and over, the same way every time. She'd have to try to learn it all over again at every therapy session. And she's not strong. She doesn't have the endurance for being active a couple of hours at a stretch."

139

"I told her! I tried to tell her 'You've got to exercise, baby! You've got to *keep moving*!'"

How many times had I heard him say those exact words to Mom in that exact tone? As they sat at the table in the breakfast room, as they walked through the grocery store, as they sat on their patio.

I knew what he was thinking. He could have *saved* her. But she wouldn't listen. She never listened.

Her tone soft and intense, Julie brought my father back to the present. "Have you been looking for a place, Mr. Bailey?"

"For Marie? No! Of course not!" he answered, more than a hint of frustration in his voice. "I thought she'd be coming home!"

Suddenly I understood. I was furious with myself for not anticipating this. "Are you saying she'll be out of here tomorrow morning? So we have to find a place this afternoon?"

Dad, eyes wide, ran one hand over his bald head, then let both hands fall to his knees with a slap. My sister exhaled—a heavy, exasperated sigh.

"Look," Julie said. "Let's go through these." She laid a catalogue on the bed and opened it. Addresses, amenities, pictures.

She, Sis, and I began rapidly checking off possibilities for a new home for my mother, as though we were shopping for curtains. Long enough? Good weight? Right color?

Julie's comments were helpful, narrowing the possibilities. "Is this one close to you? Mmmm, this one's probably full, but you can try it. No, this one probably won't work."

Eventually we identified four or five good options, and then Julie gave us the miracle we needed for that day. "I tell you what. Let me talk to the doctor; I'm sure Mrs. Bailey can stay one more day. You take tomorrow to find a place. Also, let me make a couple of calls and see what the best prospects are. It'll save you some time. Be right back."

She left, and the room went quiet. Dad looked at us; Sis and I looked back at him. He betrayed no emotion at all.

"Well," Sis said, "what places did we mark to look at?" The catalogue still lay open on the bed, propped against the stack of pillows that could not keep Mom's hip in place.

At last my father engaged. Pulling out his magnifying glass, he leaned closer and closer until his nose almost touched the small print and the tiny pictures.

Almost immediately, he sat up again. "I can't see that." He put his magnifying glass away, stood, pushed the chair out of the way with his foot, and turned toward the window, his back to the room.

Sis sat in Julie's chair, shaking her head, looking at the floor.

Mom snored—small, civilized snores like leather shoe soles crossing a wooden floor. She had twisted to a position that must have tricked her legs into believing they were crossed. The blankets outlined the sharp angles of her body. Painful to look at, but somehow I couldn't turn away.

NOTES

> Amid the challenges of each day, an obvious fact escaped me: as Mom's health changed, her caregiving needs changed. Be aware that, with little or no notice, both the physical and mental demands on you may increase quickly.

> In the stress and confusion of dealing with a sudden illness or injury to your loved one, you can easily find yourself functioning day to day, even hour to hour. It's still difficult for me to realize how *totally* unprepared we were for the amount of care Mom would need when she left the hospital. Information, gained in advance, is your best insurance against having to make hasty decisions. Ask your doctor. Ask your friends. It's hard to contemplate things getting even *more* challenging, but it's far more difficult to find yourself completely unprepared if they do.

> Do your research to prepare for the time when, even without an illness or injury, your loved one may have to go to a care facility. Perhaps that time won't come for you. But if it does, the adjustment will be easier if you've already done some looking around and perhaps even chosen a couple of facilities where you feel your loved one would be comfortable.

> Preparing in advance includes getting familiar with the financial requirements associated with residential care. Since it's almost impossible to predict whether your loved one will need to spend time in a rehab or nursing facility, it's a good idea to consult a financial advisor, just in case, regarding the best ways to prepare.

> A great place to ask questions and get practical answers is an Alzheimer's support group meeting. Or call your local chapter of the Alzheimer's Association. People are eager and able to help—if you give them the opportunity.

Someplace Like Home

*Since ancient times no one has heard, no ear has
perceived, no eye has seen any God besides you, who
acts on behalf of those who wait for him.*
—ISAIAH 64:4, NIV

The next day started with shouting.

As I walked down the hospital hallway with Dad and Sis, I could see from a long distance off that the door to Mom's room was closed. Even so, her shouts were easy to hear. "I don't need that! What do you think—I'm dirty? Clean yourself!"

We decided to return for our good mornings after breakfast.

After Julie's departure the day before, we'd had no further discussion of where Mom would go when she left the hospital. We just agreed to meet and work it out together. Attending to the next immediate need seemed to be the easiest way to help Dad cope with the radical change in his plans for Mom's homecoming. So we were prepared to spend the morning and early afternoon taking tours of nursing facilities. By the end of the day, *please God*, we would have a place for Mom to live.

Or "finish recuperating," as Dad put it.

Mom's mood hadn't improved while we were downstairs at breakfast. When we returned, our "Good morning!" earned us no reply at all.

Sis told her we were leaving to run some errands.

Mom responded by closing her eyes.

"See you later," I said, and bent to kiss her forehead.

Mom's eyes flew open and she stared at me. "No one will see you," she said. "No one will be looking at you at all."

Sis pulled her chin in sharply to her neck and frowned at me as we left the room. "What was that?"

I just shrugged my shoulders and smiled. But when Mom enunciated the words so clearly and looked so angry as she spoke, it was hard to blame Alzheimer's for the pain I felt.

Our walk to the car was slow and quiet. I found myself remembering my first visit to a nursing home. Just like today, it was the three of us—Dad, Sis, and I. Dad's mom had suffered a serious stroke which left her able to speak a bit, but unable to walk. She stayed in the home until she died.

I wondered if Dad was remembering that visit as well.

Sis and I hadn't brought our husbands along to visit Grandmother with Dad. Mom, never fond of Dad's mother, wasn't with us, either.

On that sunny evening, Dad's face looked as grim as I had ever seen him. Still wearing the brown slacks, long-sleeved white shirt, and dark tie he had worn to work that morning, he stared down at his always-polished brown wingtips as we walked across the parking lot.

From the outside, the building looked newish, plain, functional. Not ugly, just solid brick blah. Inside, we stepped into a long narrow hallway, cold with fluorescent lighting. Openings to wider perpendicular halls lined up left and right, each marked with a sign indicating which room numbers were this direction, which were the other way. We looked for my grandmother's number and turned toward it.

Beige linoleum, spattered with tiny flecks of blue, black, and brown, covered the floor. The walls were beige, the doors also; some open, some closed. From some rooms, we heard televisions; from others, moaning; from others, nothing at all. The sharp smell of disinfectant fought to conquer the stale ammonia smell of urine. Everywhere we walked, the urine was winning.

As we neared my grandmother's room, I saw dim light spilling out the half-open door and heard a low groan, repeated regularly, like breathing. Sis and I walked through the door behind Dad.

Two steps in, we heard him say, "Well, what in the…Mom! What are you doing?"

As his words drowned out the groaning, I stared at the nearer of the two beds. That half of the room was dark, save for a narrow dusty beam of light that started somewhere farther in. It ran toward us across the edge of the room and escaped into the hallway. The closer bed, the one I was staring at, was back in a corner. I remember a white-on-white collage—a woman's colorless face, thinly framed by white hair, resting against the bleached pillowcase. The eyes were closed. A pair of pale hands with long fingernails lay folded on the beige blanket. The small dark shadow of an open mouth provided the only contrast to her deathly pallor.

The groaning came from the other bed, where my grandmother lay in a heap of twisted sheets and blankets. The tiny lamp on a table by her bed was the origin of all the room's light, not much to be sure, but sufficient to show us that Grandmother was naked.

Only one of her legs was covered, and only from the knee down. It was tangled in a blue blanket, the most vivid spot of color in the room.

"You girls, go on out of here!" Dad yelled. He struggled with the sheets and blankets, pulling them roughly from beneath my grandmother who stared at him with half-closed eyes. Her mouth hung open; her right arm reached up to him; her right hand brushed his sleeve, fell, reached again. Her face…what was her face saying? I didn't know her well enough to interpret her look beyond an obvious plea.

"Go on! Wait for me outside!" The words shot out at us over Dad's shoulder. We stood like children. Or like deer, stunned, facing danger but unable to flee.

Dad pushed a rolling bedside table out of his way, and the dishes on the food tray crashed into each other, spilling salty-smelling liquid from an almost-full bowl. *"Mom, how…?* How on earth did you get like this?" Loud, disgusted, still yanking at the sheets, he said it again. "How did you get like this?"

Finally Sis and I left the room and hurried down the wide hallway. We passed a woman in white shoes, her face grim, striding deliberately in the direction of my father's still-shouting voice. We turned the corner into the longer narrow hall and almost collided with a nurse pushing a wheelchair. I smiled automatically at the woman in the chair, but she didn't look at us. We found the door and left the building.

I don't remember how long we waited for Dad to come out. Not long, I think. As far as I know, the next time he saw his mother was at her funeral.

Though I never brought it up to him, I felt sure Dad's vow to keep Mom out of any type of nursing facility had its basis in that memory. Now, on this muggy June morning, the three of us got into my sister's car and began searching for one. I was responsible for the predicament we were in. Because I seldom talked to Dad about subjects that gave him pain, we were now forced to find the best place for Mom to live— perhaps for the rest of her life—in just one day. I prayed for a miracle. *One more. Please.*

Our first stop was the Lakeside Care Center. As we parked the car, I realized again that Dad was the most resilient person I had ever met— and probably the most stubborn. Somehow, in the time between Julie's visit the day before and our visit to this facility, Dad had convinced himself that what we needed was a place for Mom to "rest and get strong again." Then he would figure out a way to bring her home. He shared this information with us as he admired the landscaping outside the wooden double doors with big brass handles that adorned the front of the building. Beveled glass set into the wood gave a fragmented view from the outside of what turned out to be a bright, inviting parlor.

As we sat on flowery upholstered armchairs waiting for the assistant director, who was to show us around, we looked through a photo album of the center. The facility was less than five years old, constructed on the fast-growing side of Dad's suburban community, overlooking a large lake. The rehab and short-term care provided by Lakepointe was designed primarily for patients discharged from a new hospital just on the other side of the parking lot. There were also beds available for long-term care.

The assistant director, Gloria, introduced herself and started our tour in the dining area, adjoining the parlor. It looked like a nice restaurant, but larger, with a big stone fireplace, white tablecloths, and lots of fresh flowers: roses, daisies, lilies.

Next, Gloria led us into a small kitchen where residents could get milk, juice, or a snack during the day. Dad opened the refrigerator and looked inside. "That's nice," he said, "but Marie won't need that."

From the dining area, we turned down a wide hall with bright green carpet and more flowers, this time on the wallpaper. A nurses' station, built in two sections that made a perfect circle, sat in the middle of the hallway.

"Let's go down this way," Gloria said. "I want you to see our beautiful sunroom. On the way, we'll be passing some patient rooms. I'm not sure whether we have any private rooms available now; most of these are semiprivate."

The same green carpet ran into each patient room. I glanced in at what looked like a semiprivate hospital room: two hospital beds with curtains that could be pulled to shield either or both, a door to what I assumed was a bathroom, and built-in shelves and a small closet on each side of the room. The upholstered chairs, two on each side, were similar to the armchairs in the parlor, but smaller. I wondered whether Dad would be comfortable visiting Mom with another person in a bed so close by.

Gloria seemed to read my mind. "There are curtains you can pull between the beds, of course, but most people get so friendly with their roommate and the roommate's family, they all visit together."

Gloria didn't know my father.

As we continued toward the sunroom, we passed residents sitting in wheelchairs parked along the walls. Most just looked at us without expression, but some smiled and waved. I hung back to look into what appeared to be an unoccupied private room. When I came out, I saw Dad in the hall ahead of me, bent down, smiling, talking to a lady in a wheelchair. What was this? My father, so reserved, so reluctant to meet new people, looked perfectly comfortable. I watched him lean over and kiss the woman on her cheek, then I, along with everyone else in the hallway, heard him say, "You take care of yourself! Bye-bye!"

My amazement continued as Dad waved and smiled to other residents sitting in wheelchairs along the wall. Maybe, by some miracle, a room for Mom at the end of a hallway filled with lonely people was exactly what would ease my father's own loneliness.

At the end of the hall, double glass doors opened out into a circular room with a wall of windows overlooking the lake. Tables, lamps, and a large-screen television were arranged among sofas, chairs, and bookshelves. Morning light filled the room, the bright glint of sun on water.

"This is our beautiful sunroom," Gloria announced. "Sometimes we have little parties in here. We like the natural light; it's cheerful!"

But it's empty, I wanted to say. Why is it empty? Why are there people sitting in the hall when they could be in here? Maybe there was a reason, but, unwilling to discourage my father, I didn't ask.

We walked to the other end of the hall, past the nurses station, past more wheelchairs parked in little arcs around it. Gloria showed us the rooms where rehab classes were held, with the latest equipment and young, enthusiastic therapists, she said. Sis mentioned to her again, with a trace of frustration, that Mom would not be involved in rehab activities.

Instead of checking out the state-of-the-art equipment, I was looking at the wheelchairs in the hallway. We returned to the circular desk area, passing, as we walked, more, so many more of the mechanical chairs, each with a patient sitting, staring. There were few smiles, no conversation. Also, no dirty hands, no spotted gowns, and no smell of urine. The people in the chairs had followed us with their eyes down to the rehab room, met us with their stares when we emerged from it, and followed us back to what seemed to be the circular center of their world. I found their eyes haunting, even the smiling ones. Haunted by the ghost of life. Maybe the ghosts I saw were a product of my own sadness. But for all the bodies in the chairs, there was too little life to go around.

We had made our way back to the parlor, where Gloria confirmed the contact information we had given her and invited us for a follow-up visit the next day.

As we walked to the car, Dad commented again on the landscaping. "Wish my lawn looked like this. I just haven't had time lately."

"Yes, that place is nice," Sis said. When Dad didn't reply, she kept talking while she started the car and headed for the exit. "It's close to Marilu," she said, referring to her married daughter. "This part of town is really growing. I hear the hospital is good, too."

"Yeah," Dad began, the tone in his voice saying he knew what he would say next might be questioned. "But I didn't like that place."

Ah. Relief. I'd been dreading his excitement, anticipating his approval of this bright clean place, so new and pretty in comparison to the home where he'd visited his mother.

"It was fine, I guess," he went on, "but…I don't know…I just didn't like all those people lined up against the walls. Maybe they didn't care where they were, but I'd die if I walked in every day and saw your mother parked out there."

"Good!" Sis said. "I didn't like it either." Another surprise.

"It's unanimous then," I said. "Where to now?"

The next place we visited came highly recommended, but it was even farther from Dad's house than the first had been. Several plain white brick buildings branched off a central parking lot. We followed a sign that pointed to the office.

Just inside double glass doors, we entered a small, even cramped, reception area. Chairs with nondescript cushions sufficed for décor. Not an unpleasant room, just all function and no style.

A woman opened a sliding glass window and asked if she could help us.

"We're looking for a place…" Dad stopped and my sister took over. "…for my mother. She's—"

The lady behind the window interrupted. "How soon?"

"Tomorrow or the next day," I said, feeling the conversation ball had been thrown to me.

"We have a waiting list," the lady said, not unkindly. "It will be weeks, maybe months."

"O-kay! Thank you, ma'am," Dad said in a too-chipper voice.

We could scarcely turn around, so we left the room in reverse of the order in which we had entered.

Fifties-modern defined the exterior of the next facility. The roof of the long, rectangular building arched high over its three stories. Glass and brick met the eye in sharp angles of varying degrees, with tropical-looking plants filling the space between the building and the sidewalk. Foliage that appeared to be growing outside was actually inside the glass entryway; the effect softened the clean lines of the dark brick and pebbled concrete.

A middle-aged woman greeted us from behind a low counter set in a corner just inside the glass doors. The walls behind her were brick. A small vase of multicolored zinnias sat at one end of the counter.

Dad gave the receptionist his name. "Oh, yes, Mr. Bailey. Patricia is expecting you. Have a seat, won't you, and I'll call her."

This room might have been someone's living room, a large living room, decorated with the simple grace of thirty or forty years ago. Display cabinets lined the walls, filled with figurines, vases, and pottery from a variety of cultures. Chairs and sofas were traditional, covered in earth-toned fabric accented by lush reds and bright golds.

I watched Sis as we wandered from case to case. When our eyes met, I closed mine and inhaled deeply. As I slowly exhaled, I opened my eyes. She smiled, nodded. The air smelled of warm sage, a touch of bright citrus and fresh eucalyptus. The scent of comfort and well-being. It said "home" to me. Not "home" as in a nursing facility, but "home" as in the place you come back to for rest and security. I wondered what Dad thought.

The facility, Golden Acres, had begun as a retirement home, made up of rooms in this main building and independent-living cottages elsewhere on the campus. When Patricia arrived, she explained it had been built to serve the Jewish elderly, but in later years, it became a residence open to all, with programs ranging from assisted living to total care.

She took us to see the whole building: rooms where couples lived; private and semiprivate rooms with nursing care; and common areas where residents were watching television, reading, playing cards. She showed us the rehab rooms, and also the beauty shop where the ladies could have their hair done and get a manicure.

Dad looked at me and Sis with delight in his eyes. "It's a beauty shop! Do you think your mother would enjoy that?" Unwilling to shut down his obvious excitement, I told him she just might like that.

In the center of the building was a sandwich shop where visitors could buy lunch or a cup of coffee. Volunteers also sold gift items there and used the proceeds to help the needy elderly.

Outside the front reception area, the floors were linoleum and the walls were painted ivory. Almost everything shone with a glow like the patina of well-polished, oft-used silver.

As we walked the halls, Dad asked questions and expressed pleasure at Patricia's answers. I heard genuine appreciation in his voice as he commented on the look, the smell, the feel of this place.

After the tour, we went to Patricia's office where she checked to see which rooms might be available for Mom. The Alzheimer's floor would not be appropriate for her needs, Patricia said. At one time it would have been, but not at this stage of the disease and in her current state of health. Most of the residents on that floor, she explained, were still mobile, and still able to state their needs, even conduct a conversation. And the floor could get loud, making it more difficult for us to visit and for Mom to rest.

But as Patricia reviewed the other rooms available, the options were few, at best. The length of her stay, the kind of care she needed, and even the way the care would be paid for influenced what room Mom would qualify for. A little voice in my head complained that this checking should have been done before we made the trip out here.

But even as I heard that voice, I heard also the sincerity of Patricia's desire to take care of my parents at Golden Acres. As she talked with Dad, I was heartened to see that she understood so much of what both my parents needed. In short, she understood that the environment at Golden Acres would be as beneficial to Dad as to Mom. He needed the facility as much as she did. For different reasons, but just as much.

And as we walked, I realized that it was not simply a matter of having a vacant room, but of placing Mom in the area of the home where she could best be cared for. Finally we left, trusting Patricia's promise to do everything possible to find an available room. We agreed to contact her the next morning.

As we drove away, the car was quiet, the atmosphere heavy with disappointment. But my hope would not be contained. "Golden Acres is perfect," I said. "I just know Patricia will find a room."

Dad and Sis were of the same mind. One by one, we expressed our relief at having found a place where the whole family could feel at home. Over lunch, Dad recited like a litany all the positive aspects of Golden Acres he had already counted.

"And it'll be easy for me to get there," he went on. "I can visit every day! Twice a day!"

We called Julie back at the hospital and asked if she could arrange for Mom to stay one more night. We thought we'd found a place, we told her, but we wouldn't know for certain until the next day. Julie thought the extra day could be approved.

We continued our search after lunch. The bright hot day turned cloudy and muggier. The stale air sapped energy from any source, turning it into wet heat.

My head ached with the heat and stress. My feet, trapped in strappy little sandals, screamed for release. I lifted my hair and held it up off the back of my neck. Three more places to visit.

As self-pity wrapped around me, I welcomed it like a cool breeze. *Too much! Once we find a place for Mom, it's not over. We have to move her there. She'll be impossible. Dad will be heartbroken. I just can't do any more of this.*

As usual, guilt followed fast on the heels of self-pity. *Of course you can. If Dad can do it, you can.*

There he sat in the seat in front of me, asking Sis how long it would take him to drive from his house to Golden Acres. Would he have to travel any particularly busy streets? Oh, no, he was sure he wouldn't have any trouble getting there; he was just wondering.

Shame on you. Three more places to visit. Three more possible homes for Mom. Get a grip.

The first of the three was another older but well-regarded home. We waited several minutes on blue leather benches, looking out tinted windows at buildings the color of storm clouds.

William, the director, wore a shirt that needed ironing and greeted us with tired eyes. We joined him in his windowless office, where the walls were painted gray and the furniture was accented by the same blue leather. The room mirrored William— it looked overworked and depressed.

But William's manner was caring and helpful. He answered our questions completely, without rushing us. Then he asked about Mom. The facility, he said, was almost full. In a voice that said he doubted we would want to see one, he offered to show us one of the few available rooms. We said we were running short of time, left William with our thanks, and walked to the car in a steamy June drizzle.

The next facility resembled a low, sprawling house, tucked into a tree-filled hollow beside a creek. It rested in perpetual shade, exaggerated on this day by the persistent clouds and mist. Inside, the common areas were dark and close, with low ceilings, but I could imagine them being cozier on a sunny day. The house had two wings, separated by the reception area and the dining room. Huge bird cages, filled with parakeets, were built into the walls at the opening to each wing. Bright and lively, the birds made me smile.

This care center had only one available room. In the middle of a long hallway, the tiny private room seemed moldy with perennial shadows. I tried to picture it with a nice floor lamp and the window shade replaced by soft, sheer curtain panels. It might be okay, I decided. Dad and Sis shared my hope that it wouldn't have to work, but we agreed that it would, if it had to.

As we drove to our last stop, Dad leaned back against the headrest and closed his eyes. In a moment, he said, "You girls can talk. I'm not asleep."

I wondered yet again at his stamina. "What are you, Daddy?" I asked him. "If you're not asleep, what in the world are you?"

I got the chuckle I expected, but shorter and sadder than I'd hoped for.

"I don't know, baby," he said. "I don't like any of this, but it's got to be done. Life goes on."

There it was, my father's philosophy of life at low tide. *"I don't like it, but it has to be done. Life goes on."*

Walnut Place, an attractive high-rise across the street from a large hospital, wrapped up our tour. I struggled to find a word that captured its personality. Energetic, I decided. Alive. Carefully decorated bulletin boards, filled with notices of activities posted on bright colored paper in large print, hung by the elevators on each floor. Many residents were very short-term, living there for a week or two of rehab after a broken hip, a month or two after a stroke.

The residence also boasted a highly rated program for Alzheimer's patients and dedicated several floors of the building to working with them. Though Mom couldn't participate in the special activities, it would be comforting to me to know she lived in a home where the staff had such a unique understanding of her mental as well as her physical needs.

All rooms in this facility were semiprivate, but one currently stood empty. For a while at least, Mom wouldn't have a roommate. Our relief at finding another nice place almost made up for our disappointment that Mom would probably not be at Golden Acres. We left Walnut Place expecting to return with her in the next day or two.

Finally the fatigue born of stress and nonstop activity shut us all down. The car, which earlier had been a pressure cooker of tension and questions, now seemed like a padded cell, holding us upright when we might have fallen apart. Silence was a sedative we didn't need, but we were simply too tired to talk. Too tired to discuss. Too tired to decide. The need to wait until morning for Patricia's findings was a blessing.

We did muster the energy to call Julie to let her know that we had an alternative if Golden Acres didn't come through.

"But I really wish that place would work," Dad said. "I'd just love to get your mother in there. If she can't come home with me and Charley, I wish she could go to Golden Acres."

As we drove through rush-hour traffic, the sky cleared slowly from the west. In an hour or two, a spectacular Texas sunset would paint any clouds that remained.

"That's all right," Dad answered himself. "It's not for long anyway. She'll be home before long."

NOTES

- Care facilities are definitely not "one size (or style) fits all." In response to needs associated with aging baby boomers, the industry has experienced amazing growth. The name "nursing home" is almost never heard these days. There are rehabilitation centers, nursing centers, assisted living centers, and more. Their services are at least as varied as their names.

- Of course, even among facilities that offer the same types of care, you will find vast differences. There will be differences in the age and size of the building and the size and decor of patient rooms. Staffing levels will vary, along with the number of additional services that may be available on site. Some centers may be cleaner than others, quieter than others (not necessarily a positive), darker, brighter, fancier, or simpler. When we started out, I thought we were looking for a place where Mom could get good care. As we toured facility after facility, I realized the positive and negative qualities of a nursing center extend far beyond the level of care they provide.

- The assistance provided by the social worker at the hospital was invaluable to us. First, she explained the kind of help Mom needed, both in medical terminology and in layman's terms. Then she took time to point out the facilities in the area that could provide those services. Your local senior center should be a similar source of information, as well as your local chapter of the Alzheimer's Association.

- I pray you are better prepared than I was for the need to move your loved one to residential professional care. I advise you to look at many places and programs before your loved one is in need. Make use of recommendations from support group members, friends, and your doctor. You can see pictures and read reviews of facilities on the Internet. But to me, the most reliable test of a home's suitability for your loved one will be your visit there. Read reviews. Get recommendations. But once a home has passed those tests, visit in person. And trust your instincts.

Moving On

He knows what lies in darkness, and light dwells with him. I thank and praise you, God of my ancestors: You have given me wisdom and power, you have made known to me what we asked of you....
—DANIEL 2:22–23, NIV

The next day was Mom's last in the room in the northeast corner. Dad, Sis, and I waited there most of the morning for the call from Golden Acres, but when bath time rolled around a little late that day, we decided to take the opportunity to visit the social worker's office. Mom's "No! Leave me alone!" was our cue to exit. As we left, the aide was quietly assuring Mom that being clean would make her feel wonderful. I hoped that bit of encouragement would work better for the aide than it had for me.

Julie met us in the hall. "Guess who called me! Golden Acres. They want you to come look at a room that might work for Mrs. B!"

We left immediately.

When we arrived, Patricia led us to a large private room on the east end of the first floor. The staff wasn't completely happy with the location because it was situated a long way from the nurses station, and Mom, unlike most patients on that hallway, wouldn't understand that she should press the call button for help. But until another room was available, the aides would check on her at very short intervals.

Just as I started to rejoice at this solution, Dad interrupted to let us know he had his own reservation about the room: he pronounced it "dark." True enough. I had noticed it, too. "But Daddy, it's mostly because the curtains are closed," I told him.

In a dramatic gesture, Dad swept one curtain to the side and held it there. With his arm still extended, he declared the room would never be bright enough. "We're on the east side of the building, and this window faces east. So all it gets is morning sun. After a couple of hours, it'll be dark all day."

Though I knew his negative attitude had more to do with Mom not coming home than with the lack of light, I couldn't believe I was hearing Dad reject the one room available at Golden Acres. I knew I should just step up, make Dad see reason, push him toward the right decision. Could I do it?

I never found out. Before I could say or not say anything, Sis got to work.

She opened the curtains wide and then raised the blinds. A shady outdoor scene emerged to replace the black spot that had been the window.

"I'll make tiebacks for these drapes," she announced. "That will keep them open even wider. And we'll get a lamp to put on those shelves. We can turn off the fluorescents; indirect light will make it cozier in here."

And that did it. Dad had a miraculous change of heart. "Okay, yes. A lamp. And a radio would be good. Television, too. Can we bring a television in here?"

"You can bring whatever you want, Mr. Bailey, as long as it's not for heating, cooling, or cooking," Patricia answered.

"All right. That's great." Still, he sounded resigned, but not enthused.

Maybe he was forgetting the dreariness of some of the rooms we'd seen the day before. Or maybe reality was beginning to sink in. Though Dad was certain Mom wouldn't be here forever, I knew that in his mind, any time at all they were separated seemed interminable. However long she had to be here would be a long time. He would continue to wake up alone in their bed. He would eat, watch television, water house plants, and feed Charley alone. For a long time. He would see Mom only here, in this room. With tiebacks made by my sister and indirect lighting.

He would help Mom eat food someone else had cooked and he'd go to the nurses station to refill the pitcher of ice water.

Here.

Not at home.

Here.

For a long time.

Though it took only a second or two for those visions to flash through my mind, I knew they must loop endlessly through my father's. On automatic rewind, replaying again and again.

And I knew, at least I was pretty sure I knew, it would not be for a long time. It would be forever. Until Mom died.

Anxious to keep those thoughts from leaking out into the room, I strode over to the window and, hands on my hips, turned to face the length of the room. "Pictures, lots of pictures!" My arms waved like magic wands, creating art on this wall and that. "And the plants from the hospital room. Another chair—maybe a recliner for you, Daddy." Thanks be to God, I was on a roll! "A small TV stand to put at the end of the bed." I marched to the exact location and stood at attention. "Something with wheels, so we can move it out of the way when lots of people are visiting."

Sis grinned at me, shaking her head. At one time, I had something of a reputation for getting carried away. Maybe she was remembering that. But it was Dad's attention I was after.

He surveyed the room, right to left and back again. "A stand with wheels. Sure. I can get one at the thrift store. A chair, too. A nice one. A new one if I have to."

And there it was again, the turnaround from despair to hope that had become, to me, the hallmark of Dad's life. No longer powerless to affect Mom's future, now he had a mission. A quest. Mom's immediate future lay in this room, and he wouldn't leave it dark. A lamp, a chair, a radio. Whatever she needed, he would bring. While she was living, he would keep life in her. That was his greatest desire—to keep life in her.

So we claimed the room at the end of the hall for Mom. Another place for her to be. I still remember the rush of love and gratitude I felt for Sis as she took charge of Dad's objections to the dark room. I felt as I had when we were growing up, and she had been there to look out for me—just *been there*—to show me how, to tell me what, and to try to say why.

We all gave thanks for the unique attractions this particular place offered my parents: proximity to what was now "Dad's house," room for the two of them to be alone, a smiling staff, sympathetic administration, and something they hadn't enjoyed in years—the sweet smell of a home.

We returned to Patricia's office to work out the details of the move. It took a while: arranging for the ambulance from the hospital; transferring prescriptions to the pharmacy Golden Acres used; discussing the costs not covered by Medicare or supplemental insurance; settling issues of clothing, linens, and laundry; and giving contact numbers and access to Mom's medical records.

By the time we returned to the hospital, Dad's shoulders slumped with exhaustion. We walked into Mom's room, found her sleeping soundly, and walked right back out again.

Rest—we all needed it. Tomorrow would be moving day.

* * *

Virtually seamless coordination between the hospital and the nursing home made the move easier than any of us had thought possible. Another miracle, a whole string of them, in fact.

The ambulance crew arrived at the hospital at the scheduled time. Their actions with Mom—swift, smooth, and gentle—slowed my heartbeat and encouraged me to take on my own duties. I simply backed away from the bed, kept quiet, and let them do their job.

I confess, I had anticipated Mom would not be pleased with another ambulance ride. Although she had adapted quickly to life in the hospital room, how would she handle another change so soon? I expected anger, at least. But no. She asked no questions and had no complaints. Instead, she appeared, again, to enjoy being at the center of new activity.

I also expected her arrival at Golden Acres to be traumatic— lots of protests from her, resulting in many anguished pleas from Dad. Again, I was wrong. As the ambulance drove up to the entrance, the staff stood ready to greet Mom and lead the crew to the freshly cleaned room. When the ambulance doors opened, two young men stepped out and kept up an easy conversation with Mom, one apparently begun during the ride from the hospital. While the gurney glided through halls lined with paintings, past sitting rooms where residents were watching game shows, and into the hallway of the east wing, Mom told the young men who brought her to this new place about a teaching career she never had and a love of dancing she may have had but never indulged.

She talked softly. A little haltingly, but clearly. I rejoiced to hear her, to hear this evidence of a calm, if confused, mind and a peaceful, if only for the moment, spirit. For so long we'd had to rely on Mom's face and her actions to give us clues about how she felt, and even then it was easy to overlook the pain and fear hidden in her frequent tantrums.

By contrast, this charming little conversation left nothing to my imagination or interpretation. It was just what it appeared to be—my mother speaking her confused thoughts with ease and obvious pleasure to people who recognized her confusion but shared in her pleasure. Another of the many miracles on moving day.

I waited with Dad and Sis in the hall outside Mom's door as the Golden Acres staff moved her into the bed. I held my breath, expecting to hear her call out for Dad, but only a gentle stream of talk from the aides flowed out to the hallway. With open curtains and Mom comfortable, the room was as light as it could possibly be, in every sense of the term.

When we went in, she lay with eyes closed. We stood around her, Dad at her head.

"How are you doing, honey?" Dad put his hand across her forehead and smoothed her hair away from her face. "Do you like this place?"

Mom opened her eyes. She didn't look around, just turned far enough to see my father.

"Do you like this place?" he repeated. Bending to kiss her, he asked again, "Do you like this place? We'll bring you a radio and some pictures. A lamp for that shelf and another chair. Okay? Won't that be fine?"

Mom closed her eyes again, but she smiled a little. A bright spot in her tired mind glowed sweetly for a second, and she blessed my father with a lucid reply: "It's fine, Daddy. This is fine."

And so it was done. My mother was in a nursing home. She had not fought. Dad had not wept. And with a little attention from Dad, Sis, and me, the room would be brighter. Cozier. More like home. Yes, it was fine.

NOTES

▸ If your loved one moves from your home to a nursing facility, you may be surprised, as I was, to be told that a room in an Alzheimer's unit isn't the best choice for him/her. I guess I simply assumed that since Mom had Alzheimer's, she would automatically live in the Alzheimer's unit. But Patricia told us that while many, even most, Alzheimer's patients do well in the special environment created for those with the disease, not all do. And when she took us to visit the unit at Golden Acres, I understood her reasoning. The large, open living area was bright and lively. And loud. Hallways leading to residents' rooms were quieter, but in general, these residents lived very much like Mom had at home, and like ambulatory residents on the other floors. Each resident had a bedroom and bathroom. During the day, with the exits secured for their safety, they were free to walk around, visiting the nurses station and other patient rooms. On the day we visited, about a dozen men and women worked on craft projects in the activity room. Not surprisingly, some residents spoke in voices loud with anger; some whimpered. And of course, I heard the same complaints about eating, bathing, and taking medication that Dad and I had heard from Mom. When I tried to picture Mom there in all the activity, I saw she wouldn't fit. She wasn't comfortable around strangers. She wasn't mobile, at least not for a while. She could push or strike out in anger, and I could imagine her doing that to another patient, no matter how gentle or friendly that person might be. It wasn't likely, but it was possible.

Maybe she was past the point of being able to benefit from the Alzheimer's unit. Or maybe she would never have been a candidate. As it was, I know we all benefited from Patricia's experience and judgment.

➤ Depending on how aware your loved one is of his/her surroundings, the details of arrangement and decor in a new home may matter much more to you and your family and friends than to your loved one. We made Mom's room comfortable, ultimately, for Dad. I think the changes we made to the lighting and furniture, and the extras we brought in, like the television and radio, helped him to relax for at least a couple of reasons: he satisfied himself that Mom would be happy there, and he felt at ease when the room looked more like a home than a hospital.

➤ The ability to keep our minds thinking positively, to keep expecting good things to happen and bad things to work out, is important at every stage of caring for a loved one with Alzheimer's. I have to admit that, occasionally during the long course of Mom's illness, nightmare scenarios played themselves out in my mind. One of them was the vision of "putting Mom in a nursing home." I did my best to eliminate it and replace it with happier anticipations or with prayers, but sometimes anxiety won. In my mind, I saw Mom fighting as nurses and doctors pulled her down a dark hallway, away from us. I watched Dad fall, prostrate with grief. Of course, most of the events I imagined in my nightmares never occurred, but we did "put Mom in a home." And she didn't fight. She never displayed even the slightest discomfort or displeasure. In fact, she appeared far more relaxed at Golden Acres than in the last few months she spent at home. Dad did experience a wrenching sadness, but the sharpest pain of it was short-lived. He missed Mom, but I believe her move helped prepare him for his future without her. Alone in the house, he developed new morning and evening rituals, new ways of moving through his days, which surely made things a bit less difficult for him after Mom's death. Positive thinking: it can keep us from imagining bad things that may never happen.

New Scenery

*Against all hope, Abraham in hope believed....He did not
waver through unbelief regarding the promise of God, but was
strengthened in his faith and gave glory to God, being fully
persuaded that God had power to do what he had promised.*
—ROMANS 4:18, 20–21, NIV

The big television screen in the first floor sitting room at Golden
Acres throbbed with images at almost any hour of the day.
Midmorning, afternoon, evening, either a game show or an old
black and white movie classic shone out on a faithful audience.

If a movie was playing, the audience, few or many, seated in
armchairs and wheelchairs, focused their attention on the screen. But
if *The Price is Right* or *Wheel of Fortune* was on, the niceties of the parlor
were forgotten. Strategy had to be discussed and sometimes a choice of
prizes was debated. Winners were cheered; losers were coached. Wagers
were made—always rhetorical, never actual—and the past and future
of each contestant became a subject for speculation during commercial
breaks.

Card tables dotted the outside edge of the big room, the side by the
windows. Most afternoons, a nurse's aide sat at a table in the corner
with two or three residents, playing dominoes. Almost every afternoon,
a lady with hair the color of pewter and a look of alarm on her face
monitored the parlor from her wheelchair parked at the aide's elbow.
She turned startled eyes toward any new activity.

The first time I saw her I thought she needed help. Sure enough, she began asking for it as I approached.

"Help!" she cried, with great effort but little volume. "Help me!"

I slowed as I approached her. The nurse's aide looked up from the dominoes and smiled at me, then took the lady's hand and put it between both of her own. With a calm smile, she patted the crooked, wrinkled fingers as the game went on, and I continued down the hall.

In the afternoons and evenings, Mom's new home was still a bit dim, in spite of the wide-open drapes. But the big purple butterfly floating in the corner of the room seemed satisfied with the light, at least for a while. Two of my cousins brought Mom the giant balloon a few days after she moved in. For a week or so it hovered, catching light from the lamp or from the little television if it was on. I thought the butterfly was a wonderful gift. I expected Mom would either love it or hate it, and tell us so repeatedly, but she surprised me and didn't mention it at all.

Silence usually greeted me as I walked into Mom's room. Usually, I responded by turning on the radio, tuned to the "oldies" station. Whether at home or in the car, Mom always had the radio on while I was growing up. It provided a constant soundtrack of music, with news and weather on the hour and half-hour. To be with Mom without a radio playing seemed unnatural to me. But in her new home, this—radio or no radio—was something else she never appeared to notice.

Getting Mom's attention in any way was more difficult after she moved to Golden Acres. She slept more than she ever had at home. When I visited, she said little, maybe a one word answer to "how are you?" or a couple of words about a meal. She was eating well, the nurses told us, and sleeping well at night. But in the span of her first two weeks in her new home, she seemed really present to me only once: the afternoon we watched a crocodile on television.

When I came for my visit that day, I was surprised to find her TV on. Mom watched me walk in, another unusual occurrence, and then pointed wordlessly to the screen. By that time I was already so astonished, the scene on the TV screen—a man lying on the floor beside a crocodile, staring at the croc's open mouth and the rows of pointy teeth inside—lost some of its shock value.

I raised my eyebrows, made what I hoped was a funny-scared face, and turned to Mom. "I wouldn't care to be that close to so many teeth!"

She laughed. Not out loud, but her mouth smiled, and she exhaled as though trying to remember how. I love thinking about that laugh. I joined her, loud enough for both of us.

I sat on a little footstool beside her bed, which put my face about level with hers. The room looked more like evening than afternoon. Fluorescent light shone on Mom's face from the fixture on the headboard of the bed, turning her skin gray, erasing even the faint tinge of color in her lips. She wore a blue and white hospital gown.

Outside the window, beyond the tree, the July sun beat pavement and lawn into steaming submission. Inside, Mom lay under multiple covers: a crisp white sheet, an ivory thermal blanket, and a bedspread. On TV, neither weather nor fear affected the croc guy. From his spot on the floor, breathing crocodile breath, he continued to converse with the talk show host. Mom and I had a discussion about how trustworthy the croc guy's toothy friend might be. I spoke; she smiled.

I had moved our conversation on to the latest antics of Charley-Dog when Mom's eyelids began to droop. I kept talking and watched her fall asleep. When at length I stood to leave, I kissed the air above her forehead so as not to wake her. But she must have inhaled my kiss. Her eyes opened. She smiled. And then one last surprise—she lifted her hand and pointed to the other side of the room. Past the shadowy window and past the big-leafed plant, the purple butterfly still floated a few inches from the bookshelves, bobbing slightly as the ventilation system cycled.

"Yes! You have a flutterby!" I marveled to her, using the name she'd coined in my childhood. "A big purple one!"

Mom's eyes closed again and she drifted back to sleep, her mouth still open from her smile.

I walked out through the parlor past the game show crowd, thinking that someday I would know them well enough to call out, *Good-bye, y'all! Bye, Bill! See you tomorrow, Joyce!* as I left. They would know me, too. They'd remember my name.

Dad visited Mom at least once a day, usually twice. He too found it difficult to hold her attention, but the opportunity to be with her in this nice place gave him satisfaction. Only one thing dampened his happiness—leaving Charley-Dog at home alone for so much of the day. Dad did his best to convince the staff that Charley should be allowed to visit. They were sympathetic but unrelenting.

"No dogs in the building, Mr. B!"

Mr. B's energy, smile, and bright blue eyes were familiar to all the regulars in the main building: the nurses and aides in my mother's wing, the administrative staff and receptionists, and the gray-haired volunteers in the gift shop who gave him coffee every morning and blushed when he told them how pretty they looked. Dad had quickly become a favorite at Golden Acres.

I enjoyed walking the halls with my father. He seemed to have bloomed here. He was known. Welcomed. A big change from the years of isolation at home, self-imposed though it was, and the constant anxiety in public caused by Mom's illness.

Often Dad tried to describe for her the beauty of the world outside her room. He told her about the artwork hanging in the halls, about the parlors and the movie theater and the landscaped grounds. He told her about the gift shop and the nice ladies there who, he was sure, would give her coffee, too. He promised her she would see it all, and she, eyes blank, giving no indication she had taken any of it in, looked back at him and sometimes favored him with a smile.

But Dad didn't take a promise lightly. And so it happened that, of all the miracles we experienced during Mom's illness, few compare with the day of the wheelchair ride.

I knew nothing about it until Dad's evening phone call.

"Guess what, Katrinka!" he boomed into my ear. "I took your mother out in the wheelchair today! The nurse helped me with her robe. We put on her socks, and the physical therapy people lifted her into the wheelchair. Didn't bother her at all! She just sat up and looked around at everything!"

"I took her everywhere," he went on. "We went past the nurses station, and I showed her the big TV. People waved to her and she waved right back!"

I could picture Dad grinning and calling out, "Good morning!! How are you? We're taking a ride. Good morning!"

I asked if a nurse or an aide came along.

"Nope! Just your mother and I! We went all over that place! She really liked the gift shop. Of course, I knew the ladies would offer us coffee, so I got some for your mother, too. I carried it for her 'til we got out to the courtyard; it was still cool enough to sit out in the shade. And that's where we drank our coffee."

Before I could wonder aloud how he managed two foam cups and the wheelchair, he had moved on to showing Mom the display cases, introducing her to the receptionist, and sitting for a while on the walk outside beside "those tropical-looking ferns."

I had not heard such satisfaction in Dad's voice in years. He had wished for something. He wanted to show Mom that he had searched out and found, a nice place for her to live. The *best* place. And, of course, he wanted to show her this place *his* way: all at once, on a grand tour, led by my father himself.

And he had gotten his wish. Against all odds, Mom sat in a wheelchair for two hours in the middle of the day. She had, Dad boasted, smiled, waved, enjoyed coffee, pointed to flowers, smiled some more, responded in some fashion to his undoubtedly animated commentary, and, in his words, "really had a keen day."

All this in two hours. A true miracle.

When Mom's smile dimmed and she began to rock back and forward in the chair, Dad said, he knew it was time to take her back to her room. She promptly fell asleep, her keen day over. But his enjoyment lingered bright in his voice as we talked. And it would glow again, I knew, each time he told this story.

That was the only ride my mother took through the halls and across the grounds of Golden Acres. A few days later, she lay on a gurney in the emergency room, her broken hip injured again.

NOTES

▸ Be prepared for the mixed feelings that may result from moving your loved one to a care facility. When we moved Mom to Golden Acres, I didn't know how I was supposed to feel. I realized we were doing something Dad had said he never wanted to do; I thought I should feel guilty about that. I believed Mom was dying and this place might slow down the process but could not stop it; I thought I should feel sad about that. Instead I felt numb. It took me a while to realize that I did indeed have one strong feeling: relief. I no longer saw myself as responsible for Mom's physical life and Dad's emotional life. That realization led to another, even stronger feeling: guilt. Didn't I love them?

In his merciful and miraculous way, the Lord opened my eyes. I saw the quality of care Mom received, care I was neither trained nor called to provide. I saw Dad's life growing, not shrinking. And I realized their well-being had never been in my power to assure in the first place. I wish I had seen that earlier. I pray you do.

▸ Policies regarding laundry, selection of meals, who provides clothing and what kind is preferred, acceptable hours for visiting, and a wide variety of other matters will, of course, vary from one nursing facility to another. If you must choose a facility for your loved one's care, those policies will likely influence your decision. Taking time to think about such things in advance and prioritize them according to their importance for you and your loved one will make your choice of a care facility easier.

▸ If you find you must purchase different or additional clothing items for your loved one to wear in a care facility, you may want to buy a minimum number first and try them out. When the nursing staff suggested that lightweight cotton gowns or "dusters" would work best for Mom's daily attire, we bought several but made the mistake of buying the size that fit her. A couple of days after Mom moved in, the staff asked that we get at least one size larger, maybe two, so the gowns would be easier to get on and off. We also bought socks, but since Mom's feet never touched the ground anymore, the socks mostly went unused.

▸ Be aware that when you move your loved one to a care facility, he or she isn't the only one who's making the transition. As a caregiver, your life will change also. After Mom was admitted to Golden Acres, I found it beneficial to step back from almost all caregiving tasks for a couple of days. This gave the nursing staff time to get to know Mom and determine the best ways to serve her. And it gave me time to adjust to new routines in my own life.

▸ For Dad and me, the opportunity to meet new people brought the chance to interact with and even be of help to them. Doing things for others like exchanging a smile, giving a compliment, holding a door, having a conversation—those things had become almost impossible with Mom. Now I realized how much comfort they gave me. In whatever way is natural for you, let yourself bloom in this new environment.

Traveler's Aid

But he said to me, "My grace is sufficient for you, for my power is made perfect in weakness." Therefore I will boast all the more gladly about my weaknesses, so that Christ's power may rest on me.
—2 CORINTHIANS 12:9, NIV

The routine was too familiar. Emergency room again. While they took Mom in through the staff-only doors, Dad and I walked through the dead air outside the main entrance. Beside the trash cans flanking the doors, stale cigarette smoke lingered in the heat and clung to us as we entered the lobby.

This time the waiting room was almost deserted. Most of the dingy blue upholstered chairs, lined up along the walls at odd angles to afford as many as possible a clear view of the television hanging overhead, sat empty. Only a lady with a child in her arms, a group of teenage girls, and a young man with a towel wrapped around his knee looked up at us as we entered. It didn't take them long, I'm sure, to survey the new arrivals: the woman looking around like she'd lost something and at her side the old man with an angry face. Only a second or two, and then their eyes returned to the larger events being played out on the television screen.

I *was* searching—looking for the right person, the open cubicle, the quickest means to begin resolution of this new crisis. A nurse from Golden Acres had called me late in the afternoon to advise me Mom was enroute to the hospital. Her condition wasn't critical; she traveled by ambulance because of her hip. Mom hadn't complained, but the aides had seen she was in pain; the nurses had looked at her hip and found the problem. No one knew, the nurse explained, how or when the new titanium joint had come out of place.

When at last someone called Mom's name, Dad and I hurried to the desk to complete the paperwork. The nursing home had already alerted the hospital of the particulars of Mom's condition. Dad showed the required identification and insurance cards. I put my finger beside the Xs on the admission papers; Dad bent his nose to the paper and signed.

Every eye in the room was on us again as we were called ahead of everyone else to the Promised Land of emergency patients: the rooms behind the solid double doors where doctors diagnosed, nurses nursed, and the unknown became known and, please God, cured. This time around, the diagnosis was swift. Mom was x-rayed, admitted, and plans were made to reposition the new hip the following day. She still didn't complain of pain. She said nothing at all, in fact, just looked, expressionless, at me, Dad, doctors, nurses. Her face, the color of cigarette ashes, showed us nothing. No question, no fear. No desire or recognition. No despair at being in another strange place with strange people. Aides took her to a room upstairs where she refused to eat and soon fell asleep.

The surgeon who had replaced Mom's hip less than a month before met us the next day in a gray-curtained cubicle outside the operating room. Dad and I sat with Mom in the chill room as the doctor talked. Mom's face was the same ashen slate we had watched the day before— lined, hard, revealing nothing.

"I hope I don't have to put her completely under," the doctor explained to us. "In her condition, it'll be better if I can keep her conscious while I manipulate the joint."

Keep her awake while he "manipulated the joint"? The joint that less than a month ago he'd repaired by inserting a piece of titanium where bone used to be?

Dad signed the form to allow general anesthetic if necessary, and we waited in the cold cubicle for Mom's turn in the operating room. Bouncing my legs up and down on the balls of my feet, I stared at the ivory weave of the blanket covering Mom. Panic pressed against my chest. The world seemed to have shrunk to the size of this tiny niche that held a bed, two chairs, an IV pole, and three people. The longer we sat, the less space there was. The less air.

A couple of hours later, the procedure was over and surgical staff maneuvered Mom's bed back into place in her room. After numerous attempts to correct the problem without using general anesthesia, the surgeon had finally ordered it. Now Mom slept, unlikely to waken 'til morning.

Though I had read that any state of unconsciousness tends to deteriorate the condition and subsequent capabilities of an Alzheimer's patient, we hadn't noticed any marked downturn after Mom's first hip surgery, and weren't expecting it this time. We thought that as long as she regained consciousness after the surgery, she would return to roughly the same level of health, mental and physical, that she had experienced in the nursing home.

We were wrong.

Though we didn't acknowledge it for a day or two, this time Mom lost a lot of ground. Virtually uncommunicative, she ate very little, and only when we coaxed her mouth open and fed her with a spoon. I told myself it was just taking her longer this time to "wake up" from the rigorous surgery. But on the third day, as the hospital prepared to release her to return to Golden Acres, I voiced my concern.

"She's not ready, is she?" I asked the nurse. "She's barely conscious a lot of the time. She hardly drinks any water and eats almost nothing. She's not well enough, is she?"

In response, the doctor who had told us that "a broken hip isn't good, isn't good at all" kept her another day and night.

Midmorning on the last day of Mom's hospital stay, Dad and I stood at the window in her room looking out on a hot, cloudy sky. A construction crane lifted a bony finger over the trees in the distance. For a while we tried to figure out where the new building was going up in this little suburb that had been my parents' home for fifty years. Finally, tired of pretending we were interested in the town's growth, we fell silent.

Behind us, Mom lay with eyes closed. She sipped tiny bits of water, but she didn't move, didn't speak, didn't eat, didn't open her eyes. She was supposed to be better than she had been the day before. She wasn't.

At lunchtime, Dad and I spent an uneasy half hour in the cafeteria. The food there no longer appealed to him. This place that had taken care of my mother and tolerated her stubborn spirit, that had repaired her body and been so patient with her mind—this place no longer held any healing for her. And if the hospital could do nothing more for Mom, Dad had no use for any part of it.

When we returned to the room, my sister stood by the bed trying to elicit some response from Mom. Good, I thought. If anyone could rouse her, it would be her firstborn daughter. Sis was as strong-willed as Mom, ready to tackle any challenge, and used to getting results.

But not today. Her efforts, gentle but persistent, provoked no change.

With concern on her face and in her voice, Sis talked to Dad at the window ledge while I leaned against the foot of the bed, studying Mom's face. It had changed during our short half-hour lunch. As I looked, I felt—physically—a new reality.

Mom was dying.

Before these years of caring for her, I had no experience with serious illness, much less death. Still, I knew without doubt that while Dad and I were gone, Mom had crossed over a new threshold. Now her face seemed one with the pillow, as if her features had been carved into the starched pillowcase. A mask. Breathing, but a mask.

Mom had sheltered Sis and me from the sight of death. There would be no visits to sickbeds for her girls, she insisted, and no funerals. I attended many funerals after I married, but every time I walked past an open casket, I lowered my eyes to the floor.

Still, there, on that afternoon of Mom's last day in the hospital, I recognized impending death.

I said nothing. Such knowledge seemed private, my mother's secret, too intimate to talk about. With time suspended I held my breath, in awe of the journey Mom had begun while we ate lunch downstairs. The room we'd returned to was bigger, heavier, fuller than we had left it. It felt sacred, like holy ground. I breathed, expecting the feeling to pass. It didn't.

While I lingered at the foot of the bed, the doctor, the same young doctor who had first admitted Mom with her broken hip, came in. He left again almost immediately, and Dad and Sis followed him out. I stayed where I was, scarcely aware of time passing, until Sis called me. Her head barely inside the door, she called me softly by my childhood nickname, "Kakie," and beckoned me with her hand to come out to the hall.

Dad glanced at me as I joined them, then returned to jingling his change, rocking forward and back on his polished brown shoes.

Standing only about a foot in front of Dad, the doctor thrust his hands deep into the square pockets of his coat, pulling it tight against the back of his neck, stretching vertical folds into the smooth white fabric. "I realize Mrs. Bailey isn't any better than she was yesterday," he said. "I don't think she's going to get better." His shoulders were rounded now, and his hands pulled harder at his coat, like he was looking for something in his empty pockets. "Her body has lost its instinct to survive. She's lost touch with that drive to fight."

He stopped as Dad's chin dropped to his chest. A few seconds later, keeping his eyes on my father, he continued. "We could make her keep going. We could put in a feeding tube, keep her hydrated…"

I had been impressed with this physician weeks ago when he treated Mom in the emergency room. My respect for him grew as we talked in this hallway. He looked us in the eye, as he had then. As he had then, he spoke with certainty and confidence about medical matters but also with compassion and understanding of how the words would change our lives.

"…but I don't know if you'd want to do that to her. It might be time to let her go."

The jingling stopped. Dad's only movement was the slow shaking of his head. He kept his eyes turned to the floor and his shoulders sagged until they mirrored the doctor's.

I had thought conversations like this always took place in a little room somewhere, everyone sitting on chairs or couches, tissues on a table, a closed door. But here we were. In a hallway.

The doctor kept watching Dad. I did also. Waiting for his shoulders to shake, for a shudder, a sound.

Nothing.

"Hospice, you mean," Sis finally said.

How grateful I was for those words.

With my thoughts slogging through my mind as if through quicksand, "hospice" would never have occurred to me. The doctor would have said it a second or two later, I'm sure, but Dad got to hear it in my sister's voice first. He could hear it as love and care, not as the next obvious step in the medical protocol.

The doctor turned to Sis, then me, as though he'd forgotten we were there. When he spoke, his focus returned to Dad.

"Golden Acres has a wonderful hospice program." He spoke in slow motion—each word came out of his mouth separately. "Mrs. Bailey could go right back to her room there. Hospice does not hasten death. The hospice team will keep her absolutely comfortable while her body does what it wants to do, what comes naturally."

Dad looked up at last. He said nothing, but the doctor answered the question he must have seen in the cloudy blue eyes.

"I don't know how long, Mr. Bailey. I don't think it will be very long...maybe a month...."

The silence stretched thin among us again.

"Okay," Dad finally said. "If you think that's how it's going to go...I don't want...we won't even consider a feeding tube...I guess she's tired...." His voice broke.

"I'll talk to the nursing home," the doctor said. "Mrs. Bailey will be released this afternoon. The hospice team will talk to you later today."

Sis and I thanked him. He wished us well and, looking at my father, told us to take care of ourselves.

The three of us stayed in the hall as the doctor walked away toward the nurses station. We continued to stand after we could no longer see him. I kept hoping someone who wasn't me would say something. No one did. So I followed Dad back into the room where cloudy light still hung in the window.

"I got her to eat a little soup a while ago." The nurse's voice startled me. She was in a corner writing in a little notebook. "While you were talking to the doctor."

"Did you now?!" Dad's words burst into the room like penned-up puppies suddenly released. The miracle of his hope and the strength of his determination were loosed in a flash. Untiring, irresistible.

"Just a little," the nurse said. "But that's good."

"You bet it is! We'll get you back to Golden Acres," Dad said, his voice softer as he bent close to the pillows cradling Mom's head. "We'll see how you feel there."

NOTES

› You may want to discuss with your physician the theories regarding the effects of anesthesia on Alzheimer's patients. As far as I know, research on the subject is ongoing.

› Hospitals can be intimidating, with experts and specialists and invisible decision-makers. But keep in mind that you are a member of that team as well. You are the spokesperson for the most important person in the equation—your loved one. You have unique information about the patient and a unique perspective on his or her condition. Except in emergency circumstances, don't feel pressed to make fast decisions. Don't be afraid to ask questions, to disagree when appropriate, to ask for what you believe your loved one needs. Your input is valuable to the medical community, and invaluable to your loved one.

› Before Mom died, she stopped living. She stopped healing. She stopped needing food. Her sleep became more like slipping away from us for a while. That's surely not a scientific description, but it's the reality of what I saw, or what I made of what I saw. There are certain physical signs that appear as the body slowly shuts down; you can read about them in a book or ask someone to explain them to you. But maybe you, because of your minute-by-minute and day-by-day experience with your loved one, will notice other changes, as I did. I felt privileged to be in on such a sacred mystery.

➤ Dad's choice of hospice care for Mom had to be the most difficult one of his life. I know the decision was influenced by two monumental considerations. One was his respect for Mom and for her wishes. He knew she wouldn't want the kind of extraordinary measures that would have been necessary to keep her alive for any length of time. The other was his belief in the concept of hospice, his trust that the body would indeed be allowed to do naturally what it wanted to do. That belief allowed him hope.

The Road Home

*Peace I leave with you; my peace I give you. I do
not give to you as the world gives. Do not let your
hearts be troubled and do not be afraid.*
—JOHN 14:27, NIV

My father and I sat on one side of a blue oval table in a room
with no windows and no pictures on the walls. Here at
Golden Acres where warmth and comfort beckoned around
every corner, this room was unusual. White walls. Fluorescent lights.
And cold. In July. The hospice nurse and the social worker sat across
from us.

A couple of hours before, Mom had taken another ambulance ride,
back to Golden Acres. Aides worked carefully and efficiently to settle
her back in her shady room, where late afternoon looked like early night.
Dad and I stood by the plant at the end of the bed while a hospice nurse
called Mom's name. No response. The nurse had gently opened Mom's
hands which lay in pale fists on the creamy blanket. Then, pulling aside
the blanket, she ran her hands over Mom's legs, lifted each one slightly,
and looked at Mom's heels and the bottoms of her feet. Throughout,
Mom had lain with eyes closed, motionless and heavy in the bed, like
fog settled down in a hollow.

Now, in this sterile and very private room, Dad and I talked to a
social worker and one of the hospice nurses about Mom's future. The
hospice team consisted of a specialized doctor and two nurses. The

doctor was available on call; the nurses alternated shifts. The team worked in seamless liaison with the nursing staff, the social worker, and the administrative staff. In kind but strong voices, the ladies across the table assured us they would help us navigate the journey ahead.

And talk of the future became talk of how my mother would die.

The nurse who had examined Mom, Janice, explained what we should expect. Her face was soft, round, and expressive. Her dark eyebrows arched in concern as she turned first to Dad and then to me, back and forth, as she spoke. She told us about the medications that would alleviate pain. She described the stages Mom would pass through and the signs we would see that indicated the body was ready to let the spirit leave it behind.

Leaning forward across the table, Janice described one of the signs as a discoloration, a bruised look on the heels, the bottoms of the feet, and the back of the legs.

"Mrs. Bailey's feet have that look," she said.

Was she saying Mom was dying? Of course, she was—Janice was saying it and Mom was doing it. I had seen it myself in the hospital. The weight of Mom's skin, already becoming a burden. The bones clinging to each other, weary and tangled. The breath coming and going, and coming and going out of habit—out of habit, until that habit too was forgotten. And the heart working now only in her chest, gone from her eyes and her face and her hands. Hadn't I seen it already?

I tried to look at something other than Janice's clear eyes and the white knuckles of Dad's hands clasped in front of him on the table. But all that remained was the top of his head and the bare walls and the wrinkled brow of the social worker, Patty, who, up to now, had said nothing.

She broke her silence with a question. "Have you made funeral arrangements, Mr. Bailey?" She stretched her arm across the table and rested her hand atop my father's.

"No. No, we haven't. Do you think we need to do that already? She ate just this afternoon…".

There was the familiar tone, so formal and distant, the one my father used to keep strangers from knowing how close he was to the edge. The edge of his ability to take in information. The edge of his endurance.

"The doctor talked like she might have a little more time."

"Well, we hope so!" The look on Janice's face didn't match her voice. Her words popped with sincerity. Her voice vibrated with an urgency to convince us that she and the hospice team would work to give Mom, Dad, all of us, all the time there was to give. But the look on her face—I recognized that look. I had seen it on the doctor's face as Dad told him no, we couldn't leave Mom bedridden; we had to repair her hip. I had seen it again on physical therapist's face as he explained that yes, Mom had done well that morning, but she needed to do well every day for a long time. The eyes brimming with compassion; the forehead wrinkled in concern; the lips moving slowly, deliberately, to keep the words from being too hopeful, too encouraging.

Sure enough, when Janice continued, her tone was somber.

"But she's showing signs that might not be the case. She might not be able to stay with us much longer." As Dad dropped his eyes, Janice looked straight at me. "You probably don't need to go tonight..." was she really saying this? "...but I'd go in the morning."

I turned to Dad, twisting my whole body in the chair to face him. Whatever collapse I had dreaded wasn't evident, not in his body, his face, or his voice.

"Oh?" he said. "You think so? All right. We can do that. Katrinka, we'll do that first thing in the morning."

Fast. How did we get here so fast? How did we get from watching the construction crane and hoping Mom would perk up a little to sitting here in this cold room discussing funeral arrangements? In one day? Three or four hours? Events seemed to be racing forward. I was surprised to find my mind keeping up so well.

Janice and Patty explained all the services the hospice team could provide from this minute forward, to six months, a year after the funeral. Janice lingered longest over the explanation of the immediate care Mom would receive. If she was hungry, she would eat. If she was thirsty, she would drink. Nothing would be forced on her, nothing denied. We could be with her around the clock, but Patty encouraged us to go home tonight, eat, rest, so we'd be ready for the trip to the funeral home in the morning. The staff would be aware if Mom's condition changed; they would call the hospice team who would immediately notify us.

I stood outside in the hall while Dad went to tell Mom good night. He was content to go home, but he wanted to see her again first.

As for me, I craved the hallway. I wanted the space in between: not inside the pain, not outside yet, but in between. I wanted alone. Not supporting Dad, but deciding for myself whether to pack my heart in cotton or lay it open to be discolored and bruised like my mother's feet. I wanted stasis; I wanted time not to pass 'til I made sense of my feelings. But it just kept ticking on as I stood in the hallway facing Mom's closed door.

From the room behind me, I heard a television program, a game show where players were guessing letters and reading the words they made. Wheel of Fortune. The resident, I'd been told, was bedridden, almost blind, and deaf. I had seen his personal caregiver many times, and I imagined her now, sitting by his bed, trying to make sense of the random letters and words.

Down in the parlor, the lady in the wheelchair was still calling. "Help me! Please? Help me!"

I heard someone tell her, "You're okay. It's okay. You're fine."

"Help me—"

"It's okay. You're fine."

When Dad and I walked past her in the sitting room on our way out, the pewter-haired lady looked our way but didn't ask for help.

Neither of us had much to say in the car. We ate something somewhere and I took Dad home. He said he didn't need any company. He just wanted to sleep.

"Play with Charley-Dog, then go to sleep."

The next morning, we arrived at the funeral home shortly after it opened. Dad's face looked the way I felt: rigid, closed. For once I didn't try to cheer him up. Instead I allowed myself to simply move with him through what had to be done. Choose a cemetery. Choose two lots. Choose a casket. Don't think too much. Don't feel too much. Don't show too much or talk too much. I had to protect myself and I'm sure Dad was doing the same.

It was raining, if you could call it that. The high clouds of the day before had sunk to the level of mist, interrupted by the occasional splat of drops falling from leaves and roofs. Under the funeral director's big black umbrella, we walked across the small local cemetery, the ground cracked with heat and no real rain since spring. The grass was a yellow-green rug under our feet, old and threadbare. I fancied I heard it saying, "Help me!" to the mist, which replied in stoic tones, "You're okay. You'll be fine."

The choice of plots came close, I could tell, to breaking Dad's thin shell of self-control. He wanted a "pretty spot" in this less-than-charming place. The cemetery bordered a street on what used to be the outskirts of the town. As the town grew to be a major suburb, the boundaries of the land assigned to hold the earthly remains of its citizens were extended past the massive trees and across a railroad track that now bisected the field of gravestones. At least once a day, trains with cargo that had crossed oceans and passed through multiple time zones still cut a loud, sluggish path through the old resting places.

At last Dad and the director located two plots close to a young ash tree. Wishing the gangly tree were a more stately variety, Dad asked about planting an oak nearby.

"A good Texas oak wouldn't mind this old clay soil once I got it established," he told the director. "And I'd like to plant some decent grass, too. I'd water it myself."

The director fiddled with the top button of his shirt and tugged at his navy tie. "Don't count on it, Mr. Bailey, but we can check."

Landscaping. This was my father's plan for the future. Found in a cemetery, the unlikeliest of places. Something to do for my mother. Enough to sustain him. Today's miracle.

Back at the funeral home, Dad chose a casket with pale pink lining, signed the check I wrote out for him, and gave the director the name and address of the nursing home.

"I have no idea when this will be," Dad said, then turned abruptly to leave. Our short ride to Golden Acres was long and silent.

Over the next two or three days, Mom rested. That's what I chose to call it: resting. Through visits from me, Sis, and many of the grandchildren; through Dad's extended stays, morning, afternoon, evening; she rested. The bruising on her feet and legs faded a little and Dad wished aloud that she would open her eyes and talk to him, but that didn't happen.

When her forehead wrinkled or her face contorted, the nurses knew she was in pain and gave her medication, under her tongue to keep her from choking. She ate nothing, but eagerly sucked water from a little pink sponge on a stick. Dabbing it on her lips induced her to open her mouth again and again until she had had sufficient, at which point she pressed her lips tightly together as if to say, "Enough!"

I had little time alone with Mom during those days, but when I did, I wondered if I should be talking to her. I tried it.

"I love you, Mama," I said.

I finally felt safe again telling her that; many times in the last few months such a statement had been met with an empty smile or, worse, an angry reply. "Oh, come on! Get off it!" was a frequent response. But somehow, her peaceful rest seemed the perfect vehicle for getting the truth through to her, down past the weary surface, deep down to her spirit which thirsted, I imagined, for the life that had dried up in her from the inside out.

"I love you," I said, and then wondered what else. I told her stories of my sons and talked about Dad, his care in choosing this home for her and the plots where their bodies would lie together again one day. Surely she wouldn't mind my speaking openly of her death. She would see it as an important event, the most important thing in her life, in any of our lives, at the moment. I added an apology for any time I had hurt her, caused her worry or embarrassment or anger. What else?

"I love you" again. And it seemed like enough.

One morning a couple of days later, Mom ate breakfast.

I arrived very early that morning. An aide at the desk smiled as she told me she'd fed Mom thin oatmeal and a little juice.

Yes, the aide assured me, she was conscious. She swallowed well. Her eyes were open. "She smiled at me!"

What wonders were these? Mom ate. And smiled!

This apparent turn toward health came as a shock, especially since, by the time I reached her room, Mom looked exactly as she had the night before. Her consciousness had lasted only a few minutes. Still, it had to be a sign of good things to come.

My second shock of the morning was Dad's reaction to hearing the news. When he arrived with Sis a bit later in the day, my breakfast report failed to impress him. I wondered whether he even heard me, then decided he trusted his eyes more than his ears.

All that day, Mom was restless, her legs jerking back and forth beneath the covers, her hands picking at the blankets. She appeared from her movements to be awake, but her eyes stayed tightly closed. When her forehead furrowed, the nurse gave her more pain medication. When it smoothed again, Dad would continue talking to her about Charley-Dog; about the now-persistent rain, so unusual for July in Texas; about how he sure did love her.

Late in the evening, the restlessness subsided. My husband took Dad home and the staff moved three recliners into the room. Sis and her oldest daughter and I would be staying for the night.

We talked in whispers and took turns wetting Mom's lips and tongue with the pink sponges. Her mouth was always open now, her breathing loud and hollow as she inhaled, crackly as she exhaled. With visible effort, she drew the air in over her bare gums, across her tongue, and down the dry well of her throat. When her lungs had used of it what they could, they sent it back out again, over the lips lined with tiny red gashes in spite of the gel we applied so often.

Her breathing no longer had any rhythm. She breathed. Stopped. Resumed. Stopped. I found myself holding my own breath during the occasional extra-long pause. Waiting to inhale, I counted silently—fifteen seconds, twenty, twenty-five—and felt the fight in my chest as my lungs demanded air. I told myself that the time would come when I would have to breathe without her.

Each time I put the little pink sponge in her mouth, she clamped down on it, now desperate, it seemed, for the moisture it provided. "More?" I whispered as I moved the stick around a bit, encouraging her to let me take it out of her mouth so I could swish it again in the clear plastic cup of water. Her determination to have the water made it hard for me to accept she was unconscious. I didn't want her to be awake and aware of her labored breathing and terrible thirst, yet I found myself reluctant to accept that her actions were purely instinctive.

Early morning found us sound asleep in the three recliners, sharing two blankets among us. I jerked awake when the door opened and the night nurse came in for the last visit of her shift. Mom rested, still thirsty but otherwise not responsive, reacting to nothing but the little pink sponge.

During the day, grandchildren and other family members came and went. The room filled and emptied and filled again as the hours stretched on. Dad sat in a straight-backed chair. Most of the time, he stayed close to the head of the bed, but occasionally he moved the chair back into the circle of observers that extended from one side of the bed around to the adjacent wall. Dad talked to Mom a little and watched her face almost all the time. I knew he harbored impossible hopes that this crisis would resolve back to the old status quo. Meanwhile, he kept his emotions in check.

That afternoon, between what should have been lunchtime and what should have been dinnertime, a knock on the open door startled us. Two staff members stood in the doorway carrying large trays. They paused as I stood, my eyebrows raised in question; then they entered, along with the director of the facility, Mr. Michaels.

With a silent nod to my father, Mr. Michaels approached my sister and me. "I heard you were sitting Shiva," he said, referring to the Jewish ritual of watching at the deathbed of a loved one.

Two trays filled with warm, fragrant cinnamon buns were set on a table, where the director arranged them with carafes of coffee and orange juice. Then he turned to my father. He took Dad's hands between both of his own and said, "I'm sorry, Mr. Bailey. We all are, everyone here at Golden Acres. Please let me know if there's anything at all we can do to ease this time for you."

The director seemed exceptionally young as he stood holding the hands of a man he barely knew. But the connection was strong, bound in a centuries-old tradition that crossed time and culture and even the stiff reserve of my father's grief.

"Thank you so much," my father said. "This...this is beautiful."

The kindness spread on the little table took my breath away and stilled all conversation. In the silence, a reality as old as time filled the room, borne on the aroma of strong coffee and warm cinnamon.

Late in the evening, my sons and I managed to persuade Dad to leave for a while. My husband kept watch at the bedside while we went to a nearby café. The restaurant was casual, not too crowded, and the light was low. In the semi-darkness, I could ignore the strain that painted the faces around me. I remarked with relief on Mom's comfortable state, and then, with a forced smile, Dad started talking college football with his grandsons.

Was this healthy? Could we, should we all sit and talk as though there were no vigils to keep, no signs to watch for, no dying to be lived through? Healthy or not, that's what we did.

When we returned to Golden Acres, Mom still rested. And because of Charley-Dog, Dad agreed once again to go home for the night. Thank goodness for Charley-Dog. He needed his dinner. He needed to go out. He needed some company. He needed my father.

I stayed alone with Mom that night. The small lamp on the shelves across from the bed lit the room with a dim glow. The yellow light seemed old and the room felt old, as though Mom and I were back in the little frame house where my sister and I were conceived or even further back, in the house where my mother grew up.

Here she was, the last survivor of eleven siblings. Thirteen if you counted the twins, Freddy and Freda, who died in infancy. My mother had outlived them all. I talked to her a little about that and reminded her of the sweet welcome she would receive at the pearly gates.

"You get to see Granny soon, Mama. I know how happy you'll be to see Granny."

I offered Mom a swig of a pink sponge, which she accepted, but without the desperate energy of the night before. Though I wasn't sleepy, I was self-conscious to hear my voice bumping around in the empty yellow light. I sat in the recliner and leaned it back, aghast for a second at the metallic shriek it gave as it elevated my feet and straightened my spine. I fussed with the blanket until I was swaddled from head to toe.

"Nitey-nite, one-that-borned-ed-me!" I told her. "Sweet dreams!"

Years ago, my mother had identified herself that way to a secretary who told her I wasn't available to take her phone call.

"May I take a message?" the secretary asked.

"Oh, just tell her I called," Mom replied. "Just tell her the one that borned-ed her called."

The secretary, not my secretary who would have recognized my mother's voice but my boss's who disliked having to answer phones during the lunch hour, told me later that day that someone had called me but she didn't know who it was.

"She said something I didn't understand, and when I asked for an actual *name*, she hung up."

It was exactly what Mom would do. "Borned-ed" is a word I apparently used as a child. Mom would think that using it with one of my coworkers was an intimate, friendly thing to do, something that would make this secretary come to me later and say, "Oh, your mother is so sweet! So cute!" But of course Mom couldn't have known how this particularly unfriendly woman would receive her little joke. I could imagine the haughty tone she probably used with Mom: *I don't know what you said. Can you give me a name, please?*

When I called Mom later that afternoon, she said yes, she had called me. And yes, she was angry with the secretary's response. Acidly angry. Smoldering. Seething.

"I'm not talking to anyone else there, ever!" she told me. "If you don't answer when I call, I'll just hang up."

"That's fine, Mama," I told her. "I'm sorry she hurt your feelings."

"Oh no, child," she argued. "She didn't hurt me. I'm not hurt. I'm mad!"

But I knew better. No hurt feelings? My controlling, demanding, often critical mother who found it so difficult to love anyone except my father was *all* feelings, *inside out* with them as far as I could tell. And upside down, too.

Here in this room, alone with her, hearing her breath rasp like sandpaper on rough wood, I realized she was still in control. Even now. During all the early years when Alzheimer's exaggerated her anger and willfulness, I remained the obedient daughter. Asking, sometimes begging, never ordering. I had allowed her to choose, even when that meant she received less than the best care. I realized I had never felt powerful around my mother and I certainly didn't now.

I wanted to protect her. I wanted a way to make her smile one more time. Maybe she knew I was sitting with her. Maybe somehow she saw that I would do whatever she asked, if only she would ask. I was ready.

I would stay awake. Just in case.

NOTES

> Hospice care is a practical miracle. I urge you to learn about it before there's any possibility your loved one may have need of it. I've spoken to many people who've had experience with the hospice system caring for their loved ones; their words have been universally and enthusiastically positive, in terms of the system itself and the trained caregivers who give it life. Dad and I felt tremendous comfort and security in the gentle and expert care the Golden Acres team provided not only to Mom, but to us also. The family focus of the program meant that help—in the form of education, counseling, spiritual guidance, and practical information—was available to our entire family, from the time Mom came under hospice care to more than a year after her death. Our first discussions with the Golden Acres team were difficult as we struggled to take in the reality of Mom's condition. But the more we interacted with the team, the more they became like part of the family.

> Making funeral arrangements is difficult, no matter when you do it. But I wish Dad and Mom, or Dad and I, had taken care of that task earlier. Years earlier. The progression of Alzheimer's is relentless, but in Mom's case, it was slow. The thought that a broken hip could so drastically impact her life expectancy never occurred to me, so the reality of her rapid decline was difficult for us to absorb. At a time

when Dad's reserves of strength were already severely limited, the need to make decisions about her funeral took a heavy additional toll on him. No matter how difficult it may be to address funeral needs early on, I believe the process only gets more difficult as time passes.

One More Day

*He reached down from on high and took hold of me; he drew
me out of deep waters. He rescued me from my powerful
enemy, from my foes, who were too strong for me....The
Lord was my support. He also brought me out into a broad
place; he delivered me because he delighted in me.*

—PSALM 18:16–19, NIV

I snapped awake, certain I had heard a loud noise. But the only
sound in the room was Mom's breathing. Two aides stood beside
her bed.

As I struggled to free myself from the blankets tangled in the
recliner, the aides looked my way and smiled. "She's fine," one of them
said.

How long had I slept? An hour? Two? At least two. I'd stood for a
while at the window last night, just before I wrapped myself in blankets
and lay back in the recliner. There had been no hint of dawn in the
eastern sky; now the light outside told me it was full morning.

"We're just changing her clothes," the other aide whispered. "You
don't have to go outside."

I stood at the foot of the bed and watched them lift Mom's hands to
turn down the covers. Her bluish fingertips curled in toward her palms.
Her mouth hung open like a hinged box with a broken latch. With the
blankets folded down around her feet, Mom lay in a crooked little pile,
dwarfed by the expanse of white sheet. Together, the aides grasped the

far side of the sheet, pulled it toward them, and gently rolled Mom onto her side to change her hospital gown.

What I saw in the bed was a limp bag, made of skin instead of burlap, lumpy, like it was half full of potatoes. The aides had turned Mom on her right side, so her left hip was up, with the bones so misaligned I turned my head away and hurried to the door.

In the hallway, I studied the floor tiles. Squinted into the distance, trying to determine which nurses were on duty. Shut my eyes, tight. But nothing could erase what I had seen under the covers.

My mother's body finally matched her broken mind. Her cloudy eyes were closed to the light. Her mouth was open, but the sassy remarks that even Alzheimer's couldn't squelch were like spent breath, exhaled some day or night when we weren't watching. Her hands, photographed once for the cover on a piece of sheet music, now rested like bird's feet on the pale yellow blanket. And the beauty who had played golf and softball and gone skiing with her grandsons now was trapped in a tortured body I couldn't bear to look at.

I pressed against the wall as the cart carrying breakfast was pushed past me, past Mom's room. When the aides came out, they said nothing, only smiled. I went back in and whispered a prayer of thanks for the return of a gentler scene: Mom's head propped on pillows, covers brushing her chin, and her short breaths still noisy, but her lips soothed with the glistening gel.

Dad arrived, then Sis. She immediately uncovered one of Mom's arms, looked at her elbow, lifted one hand. Clearly Sis had stopped on her way in to speak with the nurses; she looked knowing now, as if she could share things with me if I were prepared to hear them. I wasn't.

Dad looked weary. Weary of being upbeat, I imagined. Weary of hoping. Weary of waiting for what he didn't want to happen. In semi-wrinkled khaki pants, a fresh blue plaid shirt, and a brown sport coat, he stood and sighed and stroked Mom's arm.

The minutes passed quietly from morning to noon, punctuated by cups of coffee and brief phone calls. For most of the morning, only Dad, Sis, and I sat at Mom's bedside. We talked of whatever came to mind:

Charley-Dog, Dad's untended vegetable garden, and the hope of more rain to relieve the heat.

I don't know what I wanted, but somehow this time wasn't measuring up to my expectations. I felt detached, extraneous to whatever biological and spiritual processes were taking place behind my mother's closed eyes. She wouldn't speak before leaving us—would she? I doubted she even knew we were there. So what were we supposed to be doing? What was *I* supposed to be doing?

The afternoon crawled forward and the room grew crowded. A semicircle of folding chairs extended around the room. When someone new came in, we pushed back the chairs, widening the radius to add another spectator. Hushed talk, hushed laughter, some tears and sideways glances at my father—How is he doing? Is he okay? How will he bear this?

I wish I could say I did more than just hunker down inside myself, waiting. Mostly I wish I had talked to Mom. I wish *someone* had. Talked about the life her parents gave her and she passed on to us, our children, our grandchildren.

I wish I'd told her little things, like it was okay that she didn't let me lie on the floor those summer afternoons, reading a book under the breeze from the attic fan. It was okay that she made me get up and do something "productive." *It's okay, Mama, because the words from the books didn't get lost. They stayed with me, in me.*

I wish I'd told her big things, like I knew she was scared. I believed she was the best mother she could be while she lived with all that fear. *I know you loved me, Mama. It's all okay.*

But I didn't say anything, aloud or in my heart. I sat. I stood. I listened. I watched. I watched for no good thing to happen. Maybe that was it. Maybe as I waited for something bad to happen, I withdrew as far as possible from the scene where it would occur.

Or maybe it was the feeling that Mom was already long gone. The time for talk had passed, and yet the clock continued to wind itself down, with inexorable but uneven ticking.

A subtle change occurred that evening. Slower breathing or quicker, I can't remember. But the audience took note as though the house lights had dimmed. All eyes focused on the face etched into the pillow.

Dad leaned close and took Mom's hand, or maybe he'd been holding it all along. From where I stood behind the chairs, I could see neither his face nor Mom's, but only his square shoulders under his jacket, a brown contrast to the white of the walls and pillows and the yellow of the blanket. I was aware of his voice, high-pitched, cracking. His body strained toward hers, leaning closer. Closer. Their forms were one, hers hidden by his.

And, hidden from me, the most precious miracle of all was taking place. Mom was breaking free.

At last, the certainty that this was not a bad thing rolled over me. I moved, craned my neck to the side, and watched the miracle.

Mom had opened her eyes. For an incredible second, she filled the room with her life. And then she died.

In the mercifully short span of one month and one day from the morning she broke her hip, Mom had accomplished her leave-taking. My father was not grateful for this mercy.

"I want her back," he spoke into the full-but-empty room. "I don't care what she does—pour milk over the potato chips all day long. I'd call her back if I thought she'd come. No matter how she is. I just want her back."

I knew what it was like for Mom to pick up a milk-sodden chip, let the milk dribble down her chin and neck, have Dad wipe at her face with a napkin. Then she'd repeat the process as he fussed or I tried to distract her. I had watched her face go from confusion to frustration to stony indifference. I did not wish her back to life with a disease that allowed her to eat chips soaked in milk, but denied her the knowledge of her husband's love.

I didn't cry for my mother. I decided to wait until they were both gone. Until then, I needed to help my father make it through.

NOTES

> ▸ No matter how prepared we think we are for our loved one to leave us, I don't think we're ever really ready. Of course I had known these moments would come. In the room at Golden Acres or one like it, I

would be with Mom during her final days, hours, minutes. If I had acknowledged that reality instead of hiding from it, maybe I'd have known what I wanted the time to look like. Perhaps if I had tried to picture the scene beforehand, I'd have done things differently.

➤ I made a conscious decision to put off my tears for Mom until both my parents were gone. Until then, I thought, I needed to be strong for Dad. I regretted that decision later, and I regret it to this day. Somehow, the time for those tears never came.

At Last

≈

...For everyone born of God overcomes the world. This is the
victory that has overcome the world, even our faith.
—1 JOHN 5:4, NIV

Outside the viewing room at the funeral home, on a little round pedestal table stood a picture of a beautiful woman with a gleaming smile. She had the look that identified her as a beauty of the World War II era: hair hanging in tight waves and firm curls down to her shoulders, red lips that even black and white photography couldn't dim, a polka-dot blouse with a loose bow at the neck, high-heeled open-toed shoes with ankle straps.

The homogenized beauty of the American woman of the 1940s has always fascinated me, probably because of the stacks of photographs Dad took of Mom while they were dating. He developed them himself, enlarging many to the 8x10-inch size of this one.

I remember Dad on some late Saturday afternoons in my childhood pulling the brown department store box down from a high shelf in his closet and carrying it to the kitchen table, where he would lift the lid and spread the photos into a collage of scenes from another time and place. With the reverence due those special occasions when we were allowed a glimpse into their romantic past, Sis and I would sit and listen to Mom and Dad talk: about where this one was taken, where they went that day, what had just happened to make Mom laugh, who took the pictures of the two of them together.

Back then, I thought my mother looked like a queen. As I grew up and learned more about royalty, I realized I was right. Mom did indeed look regal, in poses that were somehow both classic and sassy. Standing with a golf club in her manicured hand or holding a leather bag that, she assured us, perfectly matched those shoes. Or sitting on a stone fence with one shapely leg draped lazily over the other, the toes of one sandaled foot lightly touching the grass.

Now, outside the room where Mom's body lay in the so-recently-chosen coffin, I smiled a little in surprise and pleasure at seeing one of those pictures displayed. Surely my sister's idea, and a wonderful one. Many people never knew Mom used to be pretty. The picture returned a portion of dignity that years, fears, and Alzheimer's had stolen from her.

I knew Dad didn't need a photo to remind him. He didn't notice how well the mortuary staff had done her hair or makeup. It didn't matter what clothes Sis and I had chosen for her. I knew without doubt that, even as she lay in the pink-lined casket, Dad saw Mom as he had always seen her: beautiful, smiling, at her best.

And of course he was right, in every way. I smiled again as I remembered: Mom was indeed at her best. At last. Once more and forever.

Outside the tiny room where the open casket lay, a large parlor stretched wide and bright across one end of the building. The tinted glass of floor-to-ceiling windows deceived the eye, showing a landscape that was all green shade and pastel flowers. In reality, a trip outside meant enduring triple-digit heat and suffocating humidity.

I prayed that the next day, the day of the funeral, would be cooler. Maybe cloudy. The service would be in the morning, but by the time we moved to the cemetery, the sun would be high overhead. The little ash tree next to the grave site would provide precious little shade.

This evening, the parlor space was crowded, but at least the air inside was cool and dry. There was no hint of tragedy in the room, not even a great sense of loss that I could detect. As often happens at the funeral for an old person who has been ill for a long time, the talk was more about the living than the dead. The old stories being retold were of my father, not my mother. Lives that had drifted apart were reconnecting. At last Dad could visit with his family and old friends. Carry on a conversation uninterrupted by Mom. Tell a whole story without rushing off to check on her.

He would eventually learn to appreciate these pleasures. But not today. Still stiff with sorrow and fatigue, Dad managed to smile and talk as the crowd moved around him, holding him up the way dense underbrush props an old hollow tree whose roots are giving way.

Early on in the time allotted for visitation, I moved out of the parlor and into the viewing room. I told myself that most people would pass by the casket at some point, so I'd be able to see and speak with everyone. The truth was that I wanted away from the crowd. I wanted to sit and be quiet.

But I sabotaged myself. As people stepped carefully into the room where Mom lay, I followed old instincts, focusing my attention on making each visitor feel welcome. Feel comfortable. I grasped for a personal anecdote to recall for this neighbor, for that cousin, for Ima Jean the hairdresser, even for my sister's coworkers, who were strangers to me. I was aware of what I was doing, frustrated with myself for doing it, but I didn't stop. It seemed I *couldn't* stop.

The scene I would like to remember is very different. In it, I would be sitting on the purple cushioned settee, staring at the watered silk pattern of the wallpaper beyond the open casket lid. I would have memorized the smell of the flowers and plants that filled the room. I'd greet each visitor with only a gesture and a smile before returning to my study of the baskets, the bows, the shape of my hands against the dark blue flowers on my skirt. I'd pay attention to the cycling air conditioner, the music coming from speakers in the ceiling, and the indecipherable conversation from the parlor. I'd listen to my thoughts.

What I wanted to do was mourn. Wasn't that the purpose of this place and time? I guess I expected mourning to overtake me, when what I needed was to take it up, commune with it.

After what seemed a very long time, the parlor emptied. Part of the family drifted back into the coffin room, filling it with a restless energy. Dad, however, remained outside. Soon, in a loud voice, he ended the evening. "Charley-Dog's getting lonesome."

Many times as I was growing up, Dad made the statement that if Mom died before him, my sister and I should *be prepared,* because he'd *be gone three days after her.* The statement didn't strike me as bizarre back then. Instead, I saw it as romantic, tragic, sad. *What love!* my teenage self thought. *What devotion! What would it feel like to have someone say they can't live without you?*

Now I wondered about Dad's intentions. But only briefly. For one thing, I hadn't heard the three-day promise in a long time. But I had a larger and much better reason not to worry about Dad: I'd grown to know him. Though all my life I had known and revered Mom's husband, these last four years had shown me the man who was my father. I had talked to him, listened to his ideas and opinions, even disagreed with him, though in matters concerning Mom I always capitulated. I had seen his hunger for new experiences. I had witnessed his drive to learn, to keep up with technology and research and anything else that kept moving forward. I had discovered what he wanted from life and how he wanted to live it: full out, all the way.

I began to see that, for most if not all their marriage, Dad had been wearing a mask, a veneer of satisfaction. Their small, safe life had been dictated by Mom's fears. "Whatever you want, honey"—I must have heard him say it a million times. But no more. Now life would be what *he* made of it.

And, of course, Dad had been enduring this loss for years. The pain was no less sharp for its languid, meandering stroll through their lives. The slow tearing away of all he knew and loved about Mom and all he dreamed they still had before them was an exquisite suffering that surely made her death seem like release.

Release.

For Mom, of course. But Dad's release, too. Freedom from losing more of her every day. Freedom from having to participate in her mental and physical decline. Freedom from the daily dose of new pain. Now he still carried pain, but it wouldn't grow worse every day.

So I expected him to mourn. And then I expected he would start living again, with an energy equal to or surpassing his present sorrow.

But first, the funeral.

Expressed on the day we chose Mom's casket, Dad's desires regarding the service were few, but extreme: no music, no sermon, and no eulogy. We came close to making the mistake of following his wishes to the letter.

But when Sis and I sat down to write out the details, I realized all the no's left us with very little. The plans sketched a mere skeleton of a service, designed to accomplish the formalities while sparing Dad any pain he could be spared. We finally talked him into a compromise regarding the music: the organist could play a couple of Mom's favorite hymns, as long as there was no singing. Although the wordless tunes would carry no message of praise, sadness, or faith, at least their familiar and sweet melodies might bring some comfort. We told the priest who would officiate there would be no eulogy, and no need for him to speak beyond saying the prayers and reading the Scriptures. We would walk behind the casket into the church, listen to music, pray, listen to Scripture, and then walk out again.

Such was the plan. But as I contemplated the nameless, faceless ritual we had outlined, I decided I couldn't accept it. Alzheimer's had stolen Mom's identity years ago. I was unwilling to let the fear of too much grief keep us from formally and publicly returning it to her at her funeral.

Perhaps Dad was thinking that only his memories mattered and he couldn't bear to share them. Maybe he wasn't thinking at all, beyond wanting the ceremony to be over. But me? I was thinking someone should step up. Someone must speak for my mother. My sons, perhaps. But no. They were too mindful of their grandfather's pain. They, with my nieces and nephews, were afraid to test the limits of his endurance. My sister didn't volunteer either.

So I asked if she'd stand up with me.

Her voice and her eyes said there would be no arguing about her answer. "I'll go up there with you, Kakie," she replied, "but I can't say anything. You'll have to do the talking."

I already knew, or, more accurately, I *finally* knew I would talk. This time, at last, I would speak and act from my own heart, even if it meant pain for Dad. For myself, I would speak of my mother.

Standing at the wooden pulpit, I wasn't nervous. I wasn't close to tears. I looked at Sis, standing pale at my elbow. I glanced carefully over the heads of my husband and my sons and nephews in the pallbearers' pew. I looked at my nieces in the second row, my coworkers farther back, the neighbors midway down the aisle.

Where I didn't look was toward my father. There was no need. We had looked at each other over this moment for years as we sat together at the kitchen table.

I wouldn't speak long, but I would say the things that should be said of a mother. My mother.

"God is good," I began and I felt his warm peace well up inside me and smile out across my face. "For so long, Mama's been lost, far away, but now she's here with us again."

I reached for my sister's wrist and held her hand up in front of us. "See? She's right here, as close as these hands. They're shaped just like Mom's, right down to her beautiful nails."

"And look! She's as near as my feet!" I slipped the shoe off one foot and stuck it out to the side of the pulpit, wiggling my toes in my stockings. "Mine are as wide and square as Mom's were." A ripple of laughter that started in the pallbearers' pew made its way through the small gathering.

"She's as near as the grandson who grew up loving country music because Gramma did, the granddaughter who loves to go barefoot like Gramma, the grandson whose instinct to give everyone a nickname came directly from his grandmother.

"As Mom gave us all life, she gave us herself. Some of the best of us and some of our faults were hers first.

"And because of that, a miracle will show itself every day: Mom here among us, among our children, among their children. To see the miracle of her freedom, the fullness and perfection of her new life in heaven—that requires the eyes of faith. But this other miracle, Mom's life continuing to shine out here on earth—we can see that with our poor human vision every day if we will.

"That miracle of Mama's, Gramma's, Marie's life has been here all along, even while Alzheimer's seemed to be winning. It's here now as we prepare to bury her body. It will still be here when the worst of our mourning is past. Seeing her still among us will prompt sweet memories. It will encourage our healing. It will be a way we can move forward. Her life won't be shrouded in Alzheimer's anymore. It will thrive as we thrive, shine as we shine.

"God is good. He took Mom back from Alzheimer's. He gave her back to us. Let's rejoice in that. Let's thank the Lord for the life she lived…she *still* lives."

That's what I said. And it was true. Mom was living again, in every sense of the word. That truth felt wonderful. Not bittersweet, but purely wonderful. At last.

NOTES

➤ I wish I had shown Mom more photographs. I think pictures of her and Dad when they were young, of our family when Sis and I were children, and of our larger family after we got married might have stimulated her interest in a positive way. Instead of asking if the car was ok, or what the paper shredder was, maybe Mom would have asked who those children were in that picture. Even if she didn't recognize herself sitting on a horse at Lake Catherine, surely telling her the story of that day would have been a pleasant conversation for all of us. And it would have helped me, I know, to remember Mom's better days. Memories of her sitting at her sewing machine, gardening, or waterskiing would have been good replacements for the scenes that rotated through my mind as I lay awake trying to sleep in those last months. Pictures would have brought back the good days and reminded me of who Mom really was.

➤ An Alzheimer's funeral presents some unique difficulties. For example, a great number of friends and neighbors sent a card to my father, but didn't attend the funeral, perhaps because Mom and Dad had been secluded for so long. Many of the people who did come to the services hadn't seen or spoken to Mom for years. They might have wanted to, even tried to, but Dad wouldn't allow it. I watched as his embarrassment and discomfort became theirs also when they saw him again. Some members of the family who had witnessed the ravages of Alzheimer's from a distance found it difficult to understand Dad's crushing sadness.

In short, I think Alzheimer's is still an illness many people try to hide, and hide from. So people who have no experience with the disease don't know quite how to react to those who have Alzheimer's, in life or in death.

➤ The days of caregivers are filled with instances when their emotions must be held in tight control. I learned to suppress anger, conquer self-pity, postpone sadness, manage pain. When Mom died, all those skills were still sharp and functioning, so I found it easy to put off grieving. I pray you don't detour around your emotions, but walk into them and through them, in the way that brings you the most comfort.

Helps

I instruct you in the way of wisdom and lead you along straight paths. When you walk, your steps will not be hampered; when you run, you will not stumble.
—PROVERBS 4:11–12, NIV

A
s Dad and I set out on our journey into Alzheimer's, I wanted to know we could do it. Really, I wanted to know *I* could do it: take care of Mom as Alzheimer's robbed her of her identity and her life, and take care of Dad as the disease slowly but relentlessly changed his home, his habits, his life.

Though I've found at support group meetings that many people want to understand the *science* of Alzheimer's, I didn't seek a clinical analysis of the disease, And I didn't want information prepared only by or for professional caregivers. Dad's refusal to allow professionals to help, along with my unwise acceptance of his wishes, meant Mom's care would come from me, her daughter, and him, her husband.

While literature written for caregivers in facilities specializing in Alzheimer's care was relatively plentiful, much of it assumed levels of training and experience Dad and I didn't have, and the availability of equipment and support staff that also lay far beyond our reach. I found that literature written by doctors, nurses, and professionals tended to downplay many aspects of Alzheimer's care: the magnitude of a patient's outbursts of extreme anger or fear, for example, and the effects of those outbursts on a family member who experiences them every day, maybe many times a day. The advice to "stay calm and employ distractions" might be reasonable to a trained outsider working an eight- or twelve-hour shift, but it's not very useful for an exhausted spouse or daughter. Perhaps the intent of some authors was simply to introduce caregivers to the behaviors they might see in Alzheimer's patients, while preserving their hope that managing such behaviors is not overly problematic.

But I needed the whole truth, and I needed to hear it from someone like me—a nonprofessional: a son or daughter, spouse or friend, who, though untrained and emotionally involved, walked the Alzheimer's road twenty-four hours a day. Someone who had struggled as Dad and I were struggling and had emerged victorious, having preserved, as much as possible, the closeness, humor, and joy of a family relationship.

I couldn't find that kind of information, which is why I wrote this book. In the notes at the end of each chapter and in these last thoughts, I offer what I learned as Dad and I cared for Mom.

* * *

As I start the summing up, I want to emphasize again that I believe my father and I made a mistake in not engaging at least some minimal level of outside assistance. For one thing, both of us—but Dad in particular—needed periods of relief from the stress. But also, from my own experience and from talking to caregivers in support groups, I learned that as the disease progresses, outsiders are often better received by the patient and earn more cooperation than family members.

At one point, I "forced" a caregiver on Dad. I hired a lovely lady, Montserrat, from an agency to sit with Mom, bathe her, and help her get some exercise two or three times a week, which would also allow me to get Dad out of the house for a while two or three times a week. Montsie came only two days: Dad refused to leave on the first day, and on the second, he told Montsie not to come back.

I should have persevered. I should have continued to insist. Perhaps one day he would have seen the benefits of having help. As it was, yes, we managed. Miraculously well. But with help from outside, I believe each of us would have been better off mentally and physically. And both of us would have been more effective caregivers.

"Help" for caregivers takes many forms and is available from many places. You may want to get assistance from a friend, a pastor, or a family member as you search out the best kind of help for your unique situation. There are full-time home healthcare workers who earn their living taking care of Alzheimer's patients. There are professional aides who work by the hour to assist with personal hygiene, perhaps cook meals, or sit with the patient while regular caregivers are out of the home. Some even do light housework. Assistance is available to simply allow a caregiver to take a day off. Many daycare services come at low cost from local senior centers and other associated agencies, often with transportation included.

The cost of assistance varies, of course, according to the type and source. Full-time help at home from a trained aide is expensive, perhaps too expensive for many families to consider. Daycare through a city or county senior center is surprisingly inexpensive. I know of instances where someone who has a loved one in the Alzheimer's unit of a retirement home has paid a very reasonable fee to a senior citizen in the assisted living wing of the same facility to simply check on the resident with Alzheimer's. And help from caring people like friends, family members, or church volunteers can cost nothing at all.

The first step—and for some it is a hard step indeed—is accepting that *you do not have to do it all.* Getting help is a good thing, good for the Alzheimer's patient and good for the primary caregiver(s).

* * *

The suggestions that follow are based entirely on my experiences caring for my mother. Of course, the challenges Alzheimer's presents are unique to each patient, so these tips may not be effective or even applicable in every instance. But I pray these ideas will spark your own creativity, feed your confidence, and strengthen your assurance that Alzheimer's is not the end of living, for you or your loved one.

SEEING SYMPTOMS AND GETTING A DIAGNOSIS

▸ The first signs of Alzheimer's are not always memory problems. Watch for any significant change of behavior and/or changes in mental or physical capabilities.

We've heard so much about memory lapse as a symptom of Alzheimer's, we tend to think of it as the first dependable sign of the disease. But memory difficulties and confusion sometimes take a back seat to other signs of dementia. Things like extreme inattention to personal hygiene, an uncharacteristic or exaggerated lack of cooperation, language difficulties, unusual dependency, or loss of interest in old hobbies or favorite activities can also warn of the onset of Alzheimer's.

In my case, I noticed the changes in *Dad's* lifestyle and actions before I saw the extreme behaviors Mom was exhibiting. He was more reluctant to make firm plans, more reluctant to travel. He began cooking for the two of them and took over answering the telephone, traditionally Mom's job. I was aware of these differences, but I didn't see them for the relatively extreme changes they were. If I had asked more questions, I would have heard more, sooner, about Mom's confusion and the other difficulties Dad faced almost every day.

▸ Don't be surprised if the first symptoms of Alzheimer's are hidden from you, but don't hide from them when you see them.

Even if you live with the person you're caring for, you might not be aware of the first symptoms of Alzheimer's. We all tend to dismiss changes that frighten us—whether we see them in ourselves or in those close to us—as momentary or imagined. My experience taught me that even when symptoms do become evident, a spouse or caregiver may engage in the same kind of denial, willing himself blind or deaf to the possibility of physical illness or dementia in the person he loves.

But failing to acknowledge the signs of possible Alzheimer's and failing to have symptoms checked out by a physician will result in missing at least two critically important opportunities. First, you lose the opportunity to begin treatment as early as possible. Various drugs as well as interactive counseling therapies have had beneficial effects in lessening the symptoms and slowing the progress of the Alzheimer's. Equally important and more immediately helpful to the person you're caring for is the opportunity you have to lessen her fear. Although Alzheimer's reveals itself in many different ways, we can imagine the panic that any one of the symptoms could produce: the terror of being lost in your own neighborhood; the frustration of being unable to come up with the right word for a common article of clothing; the disbelief at having your spouse say you've asked the same question four times in fifteen minutes. Desperate attempts to hide such symptoms must surely exhaust and frighten those with Alzheimer's, especially in the earliest stages of the disease when they are most aware of their circumstances.

As Mom's behavior grew more hostile and even aggressive, Dad and I felt paralyzed, unable to handle her anger and confusion—*until we got information.* Learning about the disease that was attacking Mom's brain helped explain her confusion, anger, sadness, even terror. And we could understand that her actions and reactions were for the most part beyond her control.

With more knowledge, Dad and I became better at anticipating Mom's needs and more aware of the need to protect her from new dangers. We were better able to control our own irritation and frustration, and Mom's, too. I believe our reassurance and our encouragement, especially during the early period of the disease when Mom was best able to take them in, were two of the most powerful antidotes to her anxiety.

▸ Be aware: the good days can make you believe there's nothing really wrong.

In the beginning of the disease, the days when your loved one seems perfectly normal will almost surely outnumber the more difficult days. You may be convinced, as my father was, that you're making too much of a few "strange" events. Dad told me

Mom's problems were probably the result of her lifelong willfulness, aggravated by advancing age. Even after a doctor told us we were describing the early stages of Alzheimer's, Dad still refused even to consider that possibility.

Enjoy the good days. But talk to someone about the problem behavior.

▸ Be sure the doctor listens to *you*, the caregiver.

When a loved one with Alzheimer's needs medical treatment, make certain your input, as caregiver, is heard and considered by the medical staff. Don't let the doctor and nurses rely *only* on what they observe or what the patient tells them. Though it seems illogical for a doctor to depend on answers from a patient with dementia, that is precisely what my father and I faced in seeking help for my mother. Because Mom acted differently in the doctor's office than at home, for a long time the doctor did not observe the irrational behavior Dad and I worried about.

If the doctor had listened to me and Dad in the earlier days of my mother's illness, he would have heard us describing some symptoms of Alzheimer's, but more—and more serious at that time—he would have heard symptoms of depression. If he had listened to us, he surely would not have based all his early diagnosis and treatment decisions on *Mom's* words and actions as she sat shuffling her feet in his office for five or ten minutes every four months. He would at least have explored the medical reasons for the symptoms we described; he would have entertained the notion that Mom was not a reliable source of information.

When, eventually, the doctor was convinced of Mom's depression and began treating it, the situation changed dramatically. We were able to arrange for her to see the psychiatrist, who, instead of relying on what she told him, treated her on the basis of what he—and we—observed of her behavior. With medication, she went to most of her doctor's appointments more peacefully. More safely. But it took too long for the primary physician to believe us. And we didn't openly challenge him to do so. We should have.

➤ Especially early in the disease, "company behavior" might camouflage the more difficult truth.

Maybe not all Alzheimer's patients engage in what I call "company behavior." But soon after I started spending my days with Mom, even as her behavior turned more bizarre and aggressive, I noticed that when visitors came to see her or when we saw the doctor or the nurse at the clinic, Mom's attitude and actions would change from angry and uncooperative to sunny and smiling.

This phenomenon occurred most often in the earliest stages of her illness and I've speculated it could have been associated more with her depression than with Alzheimer's. Maybe the attention showered on her by extended family and friends, people she didn't see all day every day, lifted the weight of her anger for a while.

Although the change was welcome and surely indicated Mom was happier, it also made it difficult for outsiders to understand and believe our reports of her negative behavior. For example, Mom's primary physician must have thought Dad and I were exaggerating her wild black moods—until Mom cut off all her hair.

The need for you, the caregiver, to make yourself heard in the doctor's office is critically important.

➤ Remember that information is power.

Information empowers you to help your loved one and also to take care of yourself. I urge you to ask questions and get the answers you need. If you don't understand what you are being told, ask again. If the person you're speaking with doesn't have the answer, ask him or her to direct you to someone who does.

Dad and I got less help for Mom than we could have because we backed away from asking questions. Two things kept us from asking for information: denial and diffidence.

Especially in the beginning, we didn't ask questions because we really didn't want to hear the hard answers. We wanted to believe depression accounted for all Mom's symptoms. For too long we let the doctor *believe* her "company behavior" because it was the behavior *we* wanted to believe in. But since we didn't press him for more and better answers in the beginning, when Mom's behavior became more troubling, even dangerous, we found it more difficult to make the doctor see the truth of her condition.

In addition to that urge to deny the severity of Mom's illness, Dad and I were simply too timid in the presence of medical professionals. *Too often we trusted a doctor or nurse to ask the right questions.* We compounded that hesitancy-to-ask problem with the assumption that, once a diagnosis had been made, the medical professionals would know what information we needed and give it to us. That didn't always happen. Sometimes when we did ask, we received no real answer, and then felt powerless in the face of a too-busy doctor and a huge, sometimes confusing medical system. Eventually we learned that, for Mom's sake, we had to be aggressive in putting the facts forward and insisting they be interpreted for us from a medical perspective.

➤ Consider getting a second opinion, ideally from a specialist, on the diagnosis of Alzheimer's.

My parents' primary care physician made his diagnosis quickly, based on a series of questions he asked Mom. Of course there were other tests he could have ordered, but he felt they were unnecessary in her case. We got a diagnosis of Alzheimer's, a prescription for Aricept, and another appointment for four months later.

But what if we had followed up that visit with a trip to another doctor, perhaps a specialist in the area of geriatrics and dementia? We might have gotten more help, both with Alzheimer's and with Mom's depression. Again, it was up to us to ask. Insist, if necessary. We didn't. We should have.

➤ "Depression is never normal."

I first heard those words from a geriatric psychiatrist at an informational talk given for relatives of Alzheimer's patients. He was responding to a question from a young woman whose father went through black moods similar to Mom's. The psychiatrist told the young woman that, following a doctor's evaluation to confirm depression, her father could probably benefit from the medications available to treat depression, even though he was in the early to mid-stages of Alzheimer's.

"Depression is never normal," the psychiatrist said. Not even for someone who has received a diagnosis of Alzheimer's. Relief is possible, he explained, for the constantly hostile, lethargic, or anxious moods that can signal depression. Another person in the audience confirmed the improvement in attitude and behavior her mother had experienced after being treated for depression.

Dad and I had a difficult time getting Mom's general practitioner to consider she might be depressed, but when we were finally successful, the depression medication he prescribed for her made an amazingly positive difference. The Alzheimer's eventually took over, but for a while, the quality of her life—and ours—was greatly improved.

GETTING ALONG AT HOME

▸ Remember that peace of mind and security for the one you care for are more valuable than strict adherence to what the rest of us call "the real world."

Alzheimer's robbed Mom of her judgment, her accurate perception of what was going on around her, her memory, and her skills for coping with fear and anger. It robbed her, therefore, of most of the "real world" Dad and I experienced. Whatever thoughts, fears, or dreams passed through her mind became her reality, absolute and unquestionable. That reality, what was real to my mother, had to be our starting point, we learned, in caring for her.

For example, sometimes Mom awoke convinced it was garbage pickup day. More often than not, she was wrong. But rather than try to convince her she was wrong, we just put out the trash. No arguing about what day it was—we simply acted on her reality.

Other times, however, it wasn't so easy. When Mom imagined the bills weren't paid or when she was certain people had come to the door to steal something from us, we found no simple actions to allay her fears. We had to use words, and they were always less effective than engaging in a physical action she could *see*.

For example, we learned it was useless to try to convince her we hadn't received a late notice from the electric company. A late notice was in her reality, so we had to meet her there. "Yes, I saw that letter," I might say. "Wasn't that something?" Then, using short statements, I solved the problem: "I went to the electric company. I took care of it."

I have heard people object to the notion of "lying" to their loved one. Personally, I believe that when someone is no longer able to distinguish between reality and imagination or hallucination, the notion of lying no longer applies. The primary issue at that point becomes kindness, help for unnecessary anxiety. Did we lie to my mother in the case of the late electric bill, for example? We used whatever words and stories were necessary to convince her of what was absolutely true: there was no problem with the bill.

Still, sometimes Mom just couldn't believe us. When she was plagued with a worry or fear we couldn't solve, the days were long and hard. But we found that we only made her angrier, more confused, if we denied that her concern was based on reality—if we told her, in other words, that the problem was only in her imagination. Instead, we told her again how we had fixed whatever was bothering her. Eventually she either believed us or got tired of talking or forgot about it. It didn't matter, we found, whether her fears were addressed or she was just tired of expressing them. It mattered only that they went away for a while and let everyone get some rest.

▸ Familiar things are invaluable.

Familiar things—clothes, routines, places, people— were a source of comfort for Mom. I think she felt drawn to certain well-worn blouses, for example, even after she could no longer tell me what color they were or figure out how to put them on. So we learned to value the familiar and use it to make her comfortable.

"Here's your blue blouse, Mama. Let's see if it still fits." No matter that it had a cigarette burn right on the front—she hadn't wanted to get dressed, but now she was wearing something that appeared to make her happy.

"Look! There's Rusty!" we might say, referring to the receptionist at the doctor's office. The distraction and the somehow-familiar face kept her walking through the door when she wanted to go the other way.

"Let's go have breakfast with Mike and Shawn." Maybe we'd already eaten, but if the tried-and-true breakfast routine could get her dressed and out the door to an appointment, we could certainly eat again.

The opposite was also true in our experience with Mom: the unfamiliar became more and more problematic. The trip to Colorado is an extreme example of her reaction to an unfamiliar place. But for a year or two before I was aware she was ill, I had watched her become increasingly anxious in restaurants. She was fidgety, nervous, irritable. Time after time, I saw her merely glance at the menu, put it down, and then lean over to Dad and whisper, "I'll have whatever you have." Later, she refused to wear new shoes and let everyone know she wasn't fond of visitors she'd never met.

Eventually, the Alzheimer's itself gave her more peace. As her general awareness of her surroundings diminished, Mom became less sensitive to new things and new people.

▶ Later is usually better than sooner.

By which I mean…Dad and I learned to avoid, as far as possible, the need to do *anything* right away. The major reason was that, at times, nothing we did or said earned Mom's cooperation. Minutes and even hours might tick by as we waited for her to agree to get dressed, or just walk out to the car. Trying to force her or even hurry her up a little only made her angrier and less likely to cooperate. So we learned <u>not</u> to make early appointment times.

There were occasions, however, when Mom was ready to go and we thought it best to seize the opportunity. If we arrived somewhere early, we hoped we could be worked into the schedule earlier. But even if we had to sit and wait, the getting there, which was always the biggest challenge with Mom, had been accomplished.

With the exception of one visit to the doctor, we managed to get Mom to each and every one of her appointments. Part of our success stemmed, I believe, from my eventual realization that a missed appointment wasn't a tragedy. The staff at my parents' clinic were understanding and accommodating. Rescheduling was always a possibility. So accepting the *worst* outcome made us calmer as we worked toward the *best*.

➤ Sometimes, backing off and then beginning again *as if it's the first time*, can be the best solution for everyone.

I learned not to read too much into Mom's move to withdraw from us and sit alone. If I tried too hard to make things okay with her, I often made her angrier.

Her withdrawal was usually caused by our asking her to do something she didn't want to do. And once she had an extreme negative reaction to a request, we found we could do little to improve the immediate situation and lots to aggravate it. So, beyond checking on her every few minutes, with a smile but few words, we left her alone for a while. We stopped offering solutions, made ourselves quiet but available, and, since she was often grumbling out loud to Charley-Dog, let her talk herself tired. Or hoarse. Or hungry.

We simply waited. Then, when some time had passed, we brought up the troublesome issue—maybe eating or getting dressed or a doctor's visit—again, *as if for the first time*. We made no reference to the earlier argument, just introduced the subject again as though we expected no problems.

Usually by the time we had approached her two or three times, Mom was ready to cooperate. We could never tell exactly when that would be, but if an appointment was involved, we knew we could reschedule if necessary.

We never figured out why, suddenly, Mom would just go along with our request. There was no magic formula to win her cooperation. It was just a miracle, every time.

▸ Watch for hazards, even at home.

Alzheimer's brings more than memory problems. It also leads to diminished physical strength, loss of good judgment, and general lack of awareness of physical surroundings. Together, those conditions add up to a greatly increased risk of accidents.

For example, we watched Mom grow clumsier as she tried to pick up a cup or a fork. One day early on in her illness, she spilled a mug of very hot tea on her lap; one leg was burned badly enough to need a doctor's attention.

Mom was unsteady on her feet also. As time went by, we noticed she was dragging her feet across the floor rather than picking them up to walk. A throw rug or a crack in the sidewalk or any uneven walking surface could make her stumble. And when she backed away from something, we had to watch that she didn't back into or off of something else.

We grew vigilant around her as one would be watchful of a toddler. At the same time, we did our best not to baby her. We kept our eyes open, our hands ready, and our gaze roaming like radar. Hot drinks were served lukewarm in smaller, half-filled cups. If she didn't allow us to support her arm as she walked, we stood or walked as close to her as possible.

In the end, it was a fall that led to her broken hip, her declining physical health, and her death. But we knew we had managed as well as we could the very delicate balance between allowing her to live somewhat independently and confining her to a wheelchair.

▸ Smoking and Alzheimer's do not mix.

Mom's smoking was an extreme complication in caring for her. Dad tried at first to keep Mom in his eyesight at all times, but he had to admit, finally, that it wasn't possible. So we hid her cigarettes and the matches or lighter she always used. Mom's frustration at not having them at hand was great, and loud, but this was a battle Dad and I had to win—literally a matter of life and death. We found that, if we could delay her, let some time pass after she asked for a cigarette, we had a much better chance of appeasing her with something else. So when Mom asked, we let her look through her purse where she used to keep her cigarettes. If she grew frustrated with the search, I discovered I could put her off for a while longer with an offer of food. Potato chips worked particularly well as an always-attractive snack.

Eventually, my husband took care of the cigarette situation. When Mom asked while he was around, he grinned and told her, "Oh, Gramma, don't you remember? You stopped smoking years ago!" Mom just smiled and said, "Oh, Harold, thank you!" And that was that. Dad and I used the same technique and usually it worked, until one day she just quit asking.

> Stay in the moment, talk simply, and speak *to*, not around.

As Mom lost the ability to engage in conversation, I realized we were prone to talk around her. I began to watch her more closely as Dad and I talked. On good days, she leaned forward in her chair, eyebrows raised as if in appeal, looking at us, first one, then the other, giving a little nod now and then, and smiling broadly when she caught someone's eye. Too often we mistook her intent gaze for a question. "Do you need something, Mama?" I'd ask. No, she shook her head, now rocking a little nervously. Relieved, we'd pat her hand and resume talking. Around her.

Sometimes she was okay just being with us, even though she wasn't part of the conversation. But sometimes she left the table. We could seldom entice her back, even when mealtime came around. And there were times her move was the first sign of the day or evening going downhill: down a small slope to moodiness or over a cliff to hostile behavior.

Gradually I realized that keeping Mom as involved as possible in the current moment kept her more alert, in tune with life. Before Alzheimer's, a wink, taps on my knee under the table, and "secrets" whispered in my ear were trademark facets of a conversation with Mom. So now I smiled at her, winked, and sometimes whispered comments to her. In the middle of a conversation with Dad on the economy, I'd take a break to ask her a simple question, like "Do you like my earrings?" Even if Mom didn't reply, I continued to talk directly—and only—to her. "I wasn't sure they'd go with this color, but I think they're okay, don't you?"

I learned not to say too much at one time; she tended to lose track and get nervous. I also learned to brace myself for her sometimes unkind or critical replies. But sometimes such an interruption to my talk with Dad reaped sweet rewards: a smile, maybe a pat on the hand, sometimes even that "connected" look in her eyes. I strongly believe that the chance to express herself in an easy way, with a nod or a yes or no answer, let Mom feel some power. I think it helped her maintain her place in the family.

➤ Use the past, even the not so great parts.

Mom's old ways of doing things, seemingly lost to Alzheimer's, could sometimes save us from her anger or help her feel secure in a difficult situation. Some of those old habits were "good," like her precision in folding towels. Some were frustrating, like her insistence on feeding the dog from the table or her delight in whispering "secrets" at the most inopportune times. But we found that even the irritating idiosyncrasies of the past could actually help us deal with the more severe problems of the present.

For example, when she was anxious about visitors she didn't recognize, I could wink at her and whisper something like "I wonder if they'll stay for lunch?" Just the whispering usually made her smile. If she was angry about not finding her cigarettes and dissatisfied with the food I offered her as a substitute, I'd suggest she give some of the food to Charley-Dog; sometimes it worked to change the picture in her mind. Though she couldn't come up with the old habits on her own, they appeared to strike a comforting chord in her mind when we replayed them for her.

➤ Be ready to show *and* tell.

Even the most basic concepts can be lost in the fog of Alzheimer's. Knowing that, anticipating it, will perhaps reduce the frustration it can cause for everyone. It was often not enough to ask Mom to stand up or sit down, even if I said it more than once, using different words each time. For example:

"Sit down for a while?"

"Have a seat, Mama!"

"You can sit down now."

"Please sit down?"

The sound of the words was apparently familiar to her, as she looked down to the chair where she could sit, but there were times when it appeared she just couldn't figure out a way to get there. I sometimes modeled the actions for her in slow motion, so she could see just how to move. But if showing her didn't work, some hands-on assistance was called for. If she couldn't sit, I pushed down a little on her shoulder while putting one hand behind her knees to help her bend them. To help her stand, I had to put one hand on her knees to straighten them, while lifting gently on her arm with the other.

Just about anything—forks, spoons, buttons, zippers, even the up-and-down of underwear—can suddenly become foreign, incomprehensible. When that happens, words don't help. Showing usually does. But also be ready for gentle hands-on directing.

➤ Pets help.

That's almost enough said. If you've never had a dog or cat in your home, getting one shortly after a diagnosis of Alzheimer's might be a bad idea. But if you're accustomed to having a pet, you will likely find—as we did—that pets help.

Caring for Charley-Dog—petting him, talking to him, seeing him live his life as he always had, unfazed by Alzheimer's—was a stress-buster for all of us. Because he offered warmth and affection without making any demands on her memory or requiring any cooperation from her, Charley was a sweet constant in Mom's days.

He could make her smile when nothing else worked. He could defuse tense situations by pushing his head under someone's hand in search of a pat. He followed Mom so faithfully that the tinkling of his collar and tags was like a tracking system alerting us to her whereabouts.

And Dad could be <u>sure</u> of Charley: sure he was healthy, sure he was happy, and sure of his devotion.

➤ Watch out for your own safety.

Not everyone with Alzheimer's experiences paranoia and extreme anger as Mom did. But the disease is notorious for stealing a person's judgment and inhibitions. Several people in support group meetings shared stories of a loved one becoming hostile and physically aggressive. Of those patients who are likely to strike out at someone or something, some are surely stronger than my mother was and could pose more of a risk to caretakers.

Mom never hurt herself or my father, but I feared she might. Though she wasn't strong, I knew she could push Dad down if she caught him unaware. She could hit his glasses, throw something at him, or even intentionally set something on fire with a cigarette. The only defense we had against her doing something violent was to be with her, watch her closely when she was angry, and stop her if it became necessary. Eventually, of course, her frail physical condition controlled her actions more effectively than any efforts we exerted.

We were successful in restraining Mom's actions when her emotions were out of control. But I emphasize: <u>we</u> were successful, <u>Dad and I together</u>. If I hadn't been there with him, I'm not sure Dad would always have had the patience and presence of mind to handle her emotional outbursts before they escalated to physical action.

I am sorry to bring up the possibility of a loved one trying to hurt you while you are caring for her. I know the pain of being told, "Don't take it personally...it's the disease, not her..." and the difficulty of implementing that advice. Most of all, I pray this is a subject you never have to deal with. But if you fear the one you are caring for *might* hurt you, take your fear seriously. Be prepared. Get advice right away. If your physician can't provide timely information and advice, call the Alzheimer's Association or your local senior citizens' center. And never hesitate to call 911 if necessary.

▸ Don't stop living.

Dad and I learned it was okay—even necessary— that we do, sometimes, exactly what we wanted to do, even if those activities didn't make Mom happy. But it was a hard lesson, not easily grasped by either of us.

At first, we were convinced we could make Mom feel better by focusing our care and attention on her every wish and whim. So if she was happy with us sitting beside her at the table, we sat. If she was unhappy sitting with only me when Dad went outside to tend to flowers or take a walk or just be alone for a while, he didn't do those things.

But living that way wasn't real life for any of us. Try as we might, Dad and I couldn't control Mom's moods; we could only make ourselves miserable trying. Mom was withdrawing from life; she had no choice in the matter. What Dad and I finally recognized was that we were trying to live *her* life *with her*, so we were shrinking, too.

Dreams, plans, projects, those activities that keep us mentally and physically healthy—we needed them. Otherwise, Alzheimer's would thrust us all into depression, and Mom would have no one to help her stay in the family. Our unmitigated grief and unrelieved exhaustion did Mom harm, not good.

So we stepped back into life. We chose times and locations for our projects that let us be certain Mom was physically comfortable and safe, and we helped her be as happy as she could while we took care of ourselves. If we had engaged a helper to stay with her for regularly scheduled periods of time, life would have been easier for all of us. But we managed. Slowly, we managed to live and grow and accomplish things again. Life became brighter for all of us, Mom included.

Maybe you think Alzheimer's has made some of your plans impossible. Please don't abandon them without first trying to adjust them. And get help. Making time for yourself is one of the most important reasons to bring in outside help.

GETTING ALONG IN PUBLIC

> Go familiar places; do familiar things.

Getting out of the house was good for Mom. I think the sensory stimulation kept her more alert and more in the present moment. But gradually, new places became too stressful for her. Unable to process all the new information, she became nervous and uncomfortable. So, as far as possible, we stuck to the places she had known and enjoyed before Alzheimer's, like the grocery store, certain restaurants, the post office.

> When it comes to clothes, concentrate on function, not fashion.

Perhaps the one you care for will accept whatever clothing you think best, but if not, rest assured that life goes on even if socks don't match. Even if the only acceptable shoes have green shamrocks on them. Even if the sweater has a hole in it or the blouse is striped and the slacks are plaid.

In the beginning, I was embarrassed by Mom's appearance: her hair, her clothes, the state of her hygiene. Would people think I didn't care about her? Or, to get to the heart of the matter, would people judge me by my mother's appearance?

I'm not sure when the embarrassment began to wear off. Perhaps when I realized that the dilemma facing us was *not* whether Mom would cooperate and wear clean, attractive clothing but rather would she leave the house or stay cooped up inside? Would she get some exercise, see different things, or stay at home because I worried she didn't look good enough?

Of course it was a wonderful thing for Mom to be smiling in the middle of the stuffed animals in the toy department or smelling the fresh fruit in the grocery store or savoring a doughnut in the coffee shop. We delighted at her joy in seeing holiday decorations, rain on the street, or someone walking their dog as we drove by. Soon enough these benefits far outweighed my concern about her appearance. I learned to concentrate on her, watch her, enjoy her, and protect her, instead of wondering what other people saw or thought.

> Be alert for potential problems or obstacles.

I turned my internal radar up to high when we were out with Mom. Of course I watched for physical obstacles that might make her stumble, but I also looked out for situations that would have caught her attention when she was healthy. A loud or crying child, for example. Once Alzheimer's had taken away her ability to choose what she should react to and what she should ignore, she was likely to fuss at a stranger's child as if it were her own.

The solution was simply to steer away from such potential problems when possible. When it wasn't possible to avoid them, distractions were helpful: a whispered "secret" or asking her for a tissue usually worked with Mom until we could walk away.

> Moods change faster than the weather.

The mercurial mood changes Mom went through at home happened also, though not as often, when we were out. If she was angry or uncooperative at home, chances are we didn't attempt to go anywhere until she was more relaxed. But sometimes the sunny-day face she wore as we started out in the car turned suddenly stormy—in the store, at the restaurant, wherever we happened to be.

If we could determine the cause, we eliminated it. Obviously, if we couldn't find the cause, the situation was much more difficult. Maybe Mom was complaining loudly about a problem she had imagined, or banging her hand on the shopping cart in irritation at something she couldn't name. At times like that, we found movement was the best solution. We kept her walking, usually toward the exit, and gradually the physical effort of moving, I believe, left her with no energy to continue her tirade.

But I feared those occurrences. I feared Mom would get so far out of control, she would draw a crowd. I dreaded the possibility a store manager would ask if he needed to call an ambulance. I pictured people complaining, children crying, or Mom getting louder, maybe even striking out at us or others as we tried to get her to the car. That's what I imagined, especially during the time before medication helped with her depression.

But those things never happened. For one thing, Dad and I had the distinct advantage of working as a team: two heads, two mouths, and four hands. In addition, I never took Mom's good moods for granted. I was always watchful: for signs she was getting tired, for unusual situations that might frighten her, for the furrowed brow or tight lips that warned of her irritation. We knew what to do: one of us kept her moving toward the car and the other finished whatever business, if any, was being conducted. As at home, we kept our reactions low-key, our words casual.

The public catastrophes never came about. And even my fears diminished over time, as I realized we were capable, assistance would always be available, and people were kinder and more helpful than I had ever realized.

> Prepare to be amazed and comforted by the kindness of strangers.

If Mom's appearance or actions ever prompted amused looks or unkind comments, I never saw or heard them. Heaven's protection played a part in that, I know, but I think also that people are nicer than my pre-Alzheimer's consciousness realized. I came to expect people to be kind to Mom. Most were. I began to expect people to understand her condition without having it explained. Most did.

> Let people help.

It's natural to try to keep up appearances. As Dad and I tried to keep life as normal as possible, we sought to make our errand-running threesome blend into the public scene. But that became difficult, then harder, and finally impossible. People saw. They heard. They knew.

But, wonder of wonders, when we needed help, they helped, with sweet miracles, large and small, depending on the level of our need. We found it hard to accept their kindness at first. For me it was concern with appearances again, I suppose. As for Dad, his reluctance to accept help came from two sources: one, his steadfast determination that *he* was all the help Mom needed, and two, his quest for privacy that so often put blinders on his eyes. He was blind to his own need and blind to offers of assistance that came his way. I was embarrassed, and he was blind. Both of us too proud.

Gradually, miraculously, we learned. Well, mostly I learned. Dad often looked the other way when someone offered to help with a shopping cart or made a path for him as Mom shuffled alongside. But finally I put down my embarrassment and faced the truth. Oh, I waited as long as I could—until reality was forced on me, until I could no longer shut my eyes to the truth of Mom's difficulties and the sometimes overwhelming burden they put on me and Dad. But who was I, I finally realized, to decide that people who said they'd be glad to help were just being polite or nice? I could trust them to speak their own truth. Not quickly, but eventually, I surrendered. I learned to trust, and to welcome the assistance of friends and strangers alike.

I pray you will, too. People who have nothing to gain, people who have other responsibilities, people you know not at all, just plain nice people will help by giving you a place up front in a long line or by saying "hello" to the person you're caring for when she speaks to them or by taking your cart inside so you can help her remember how to sit down in the car. People like Mike and Shaun will do bigger favors for you than you can ever hope to repay.

Just let it happen. Let people give. Learn to accept. You'll be better for it, and so will they.

HYGIENE AND EXERCISE

▶ Establish a "clean routine" early on.

The earlier the better! I wish I had. By the time I stepped in to help with Mom's daily care, she was already very reluctant to bathe, brush her teeth, and even wash her hands. She was such a fanatic about cleanliness when I was growing up, I could scarcely believe Alzheimer's would make her flatly refuse to wash her hands before a meal. And Dad wasn't much help in this area. Thinking he was choosing his battles wisely, he saved his strongest efforts for getting Mom to take her medicine and eat regularly. He wouldn't challenge her when she said she "bathed yesterday" or washed her hands "a few minutes ago." His bad eyesight multiplied the difficulties, since he couldn't see how badly she needed to wash.

Some willfulness was involved in Mom's refusal to bathe, especially early on, but the decline of her mental and physical capabilities made proper hygiene a tremendous problem. And so it is with many Alzheimer's patients: just getting dressed and undressed comes to be a challenge. The movements which for most of us are instinctive—not just buttoning and unbuttoning, but moving an arm in the proper direction to get it out of a sleeve or lifting a leg to put on underwear, slacks, socks, and shoes—those movements become a greater and greater ordeal for the Alzheimer's patient, both physically and mentally. So they do what's natural—they resist.

Before Mom's mind lost the notion of being clean, I wish I'd made bath time and "beauty shop" time an appointment for fun with her. Even before my help became necessary for her safety, I wish I'd joined her in the bathroom, at the same time of day, once a week, every week. Maybe I'd have played the radio and brought her a plastic cup of lemonade in the summer or lukewarm cocoa in the winter while she soaked in the tub. Perhaps then the idea of bath time and the accompanying activities—music, girl talk, a snack— would have remained a positive stimulation for her. If I had established a routine, practiced and followed it faithfully from the earliest time possible, I believe the chances are greater she would have reacted better, even after her mind forgot the routine.

As it was, bathing Mom became such a struggle that we could manage it only about once a month. Between baths, I took every opportunity to wash her hands, her face, wherever I could reach, with a warm washcloth. But the places I couldn't get to were the places that most needed soap and water. She often sat in wet or soiled underwear for hours at a time. When she finally allowed me to tend to it, I cleaned everything as best I could without getting her into a tub or shower. I did what was possible and, by the daily miracles that always saved us, it was enough. Mom never developed even a skin rash. Her doctors were satisfied with her level of cleanliness. But a routine would almost certainly have kept her cleaner and more comfortable.

Another note: bathing an adult isn't easy. If you consider getting professional help even on a very limited basis, bathing, or hygiene in general, is the first need I would address. For example, I heard from many people at support group meetings that, in cases where someone is reluctant to be seen naked, an aide is often accepted more easily than a family member. Mom and I didn't have issues of shyness; she didn't mind me seeing her undressed. *But by far the greater issue is safety.* Helping Mom move around and keeping her stable when she was wet required strength and expertise. A professional caretaker would have made bath time much safer for Mom and easier for both of us.

> Dentures require special handling.

If the person you care for wears dentures, find out how to tend to them or be certain your professional helper knows how. And be ready for the time when you must put the dentures aside and serve softer food. Dad helped Mom with her dentures for as long as he could, but when he could no longer see well enough, I had to learn quickly about adhesive and soaking mixtures and proper positioning. But the time came when Mom would no longer let me put my fingers in her mouth. So the teeth stayed in, unbrushed and loose, for months. I was worried they would make her sick. Miraculously, she was fine.

Fine, that is, until the day Dad told me with a look of concern on his face that Mom couldn't chew. Perhaps because she was in pain, she opened her mouth readily at my request. To my shock, her dentures were in upside down. The teeth surfaces were against her gums. I don't know how she could speak, but she did, insisting the teeth were fine. Except for doing what teeth were intended to do: chew.

Bottom line: watch out for dentures. Though her appearance suffered and her food choices were narrowed, Mom was finally better off without hers.

> Prepare in advance for incontinence.

Disposable underwear products are miracles. They are made in at least two varieties: the kind that opens on each side (easy to change, especially for those who are bedridden) and the pull-up variety, which also opens on the sides. Both kinds are super absorbent and the fit has been designed to give excellent protection.

Washable waterproof mattress pads are good insurance. They go under the bed sheet and cover the entire mattress.

Disposable waterproof pads can be placed on top of the sheet to eliminate the need to wash bedclothes every day. The pads will also protect car seats and furniture.

In addition to the items we used in the house, when we went out somewhere, I always had wipes, underwear, and a change of clothes for Mom in case of an emergency. We never needed them, but we were prepared, just in case.

Mom continued to insist for a long time that she didn't need disposable underwear. Strong evidence indicated otherwise. When persuasion didn't work, we got rid of all her other underwear, leaving only disposables in her drawer. Always resourceful, Mom began wearing Dad's boxers. So he hid them from her, stashing them in a desk drawer. And, thank goodness, my mother preferred wearing disposables to going without. The value of a good old-fashioned upbringing cannot be overestimated.

One more thing: perhaps neither you, nor the one you care for is offended by use of the term "diapers" to refer to disposable underwear for adults. I was. Out of respect for my mother, I never used that word.

▸ Exercise is still possible and still beneficial.

Of course the first thing that must be said about exercise is that a physician is the one to determine the healthiest type and level of physical activity for the one you are caring for.

In Mom's case, her reluctance to engage in any kind of physical activity was one of the first signs to Dad that she was ill. Such reluctance is common for those with Alzheimer's, but we knew that keeping Mom mobile for as long as possible was good for her. So we encouraged her to walk with us. Alas, even short, slow walks upset her, especially if we were outside. One day, however, we realized Mom would walk happily behind a cart in the grocery store. Her gait grew more unsteady as time passed, and she wouldn't use a cane or a walker, but she leaned on the grocery cart and let it take her on long, slow tours of the store.

Of course we should also note that people with Alzheimer's are as unique after they have the disease as they were before. So they will have their own ways of getting exercise, at least in the earlier stages. Some will dance. Some will garden. Some will walk or shoot baskets. Mom got her exercise on our shopping trips. With extra attention to safety, such activities can be a continuing and familiar source of health and fun for a long time.

LEGAL MATTERS

We waited almost too late to get Mom's signature on the durable power of attorney. Only by a miracle did she convince the notary that she understood what she was signing. Only by a miracle was she able to sign her name. There were many things Mom couldn't understand or couldn't do, but on that particular day, she could do what was needed.

Legal matters must be handled while your loved one can still make sensible decisions for herself. A will and a durable power of attorney (one which specifically states that it can be exercised even if the person becomes mentally incapacitated) are the documents we heard about most often from doctors and at support group meetings. My parents had made their wills many years before. Their estate was a simple one, which required no updating. But Mom's signature on the durable power of attorney eliminated the necessity of going to court to handle the decisions and take the actions she was eventually incapable of handling. If Dad had died before her, the power of attorney would have been all the more important.

A lawyer is the best authority on the legal matters associated with your loved one's growing mental disability. The Alzheimer's Association and your local senior citizens agency can also give you information regarding the laws and practices that pertain to you in your state. There is no easier time than the present to attend to these matters.

THE THINGS WE DIDN'T HAVE TO DEAL WITH, AND THE MOST IMPORTANT HELPS

Alzheimer's wears a different face in every home. Just as many Alzheimer's patients do not suffer from depression or do not become as angry and hostile as Mom, so she didn't experience some of the other symptoms often associated with the disease.

Mom wasn't inclined to wander away from the house. She didn't imagine people were stealing from her, so she didn't hide things. She slept well at night. And, perhaps most mercifully for Dad, she never totally forgot that he was a part of her life. She never feared him.

I can't give you suggestions about dealing with those issues, not, that is, suggestions based on our experience with my mother. But I can tell you that the three biggest lessons I learned as we cared for my mother will surely apply to *whatever* situations you face on your journey through Alzheimer's. They are these:

➤ *You always have options.*

There will always be more than one way to accomplish what you need to accomplish. You may not be able to see all the possibilities, but they are there, like different routes on a map that lead to the same destination.

I was blind to options at the outset of our journey through Alzheimer's. At that time, I was convinced there was only one way to accomplish any task having to do with Mom's care: my father's way. Sometimes his way seemed fine. Often it looked unreasonable, but doable. Sometimes it was impossible, but I tried anyway.

For example, Dad's way of keeping my mother safe while she was smoking was for one of us to be with her every minute. A completely unrealistic solution to a serious problem. But for over fifty years, Mom always had cigarettes at hand. Now, as Dad tried to keep everything as "normal" as possible, the thought of taking cigarettes away from her was an option he never considered. And since I was deferring to him at every turn, the idea never occurred to me—until perhaps the hundredth time my husband expressed concern over stories of Mom dropping lit cigarettes. This time, he added a question: why were they available to her?

"Because she's always had them," was the only answer I could come up with. The question itself was a surprise to me, so tightly were my eyes closed to the notion of choices.

Finding the best way to accomplish what we needed to do required, first, that we *open our eyes to all the possibilities.* The journey through Alzheimer's is difficult. I pray you will search for all the available routes to make the path easier for your loved one and for you. If you can't see all the roads yourself, ask someone you trust to help you find them.

➤ *Be ready to laugh.*

The day Mom broke her hip was a long, difficult day. It stretched from early in the morning, when she fell, to almost midnight, when she was finally in the emergency room and we were waiting for a diagnosis. Dad, Sis, and I stood around the bed in the icy examining room and waited for the return of the young doctor who had ordered and was now reading, we hoped, Mom's x-rays. She lay silent under two blankets, sometimes staring at the ceiling, sometimes with eyes tightly closed.

We stood, paced, or sat on frigid metal stools until nerves and the cold drove us to move around some more. We listened to our stomachs growling, an occasional ambulance, conversations among other patients just outside the door, my father jingling his change. Hours passed.

Finally the doctor returned. He walked to the bed and gently took Mom's hand. He looked kindly down into her closed eyes. When he spoke, his words were soft and slow, probably to keep from startling her out of sleep. I was immensely grateful for his careful manner in this place that was dedicated to speed and accuracy and moving patients through the system.

"Mrs. Bailey, how old are you?" he asked.

While I tried to remember whether Alzheimer's was spelled out clearly enough on the long information sheet we had filled out, I watched Mom's eyes fly open, then narrow to dark slits. Her brows came together.

Someone was in for it.

"Wellll, Doctor," she said, more clearly than she had spoken in weeks. "How much money do you make?"

The doctor stood speechless for a couple of seconds. Dad looked panic-stricken at first, then started to giggle. Soon we were all red-faced and laughing, all except Mom, who was pale and clearly incensed.

"Touché, Mrs. Bailey," the doctor said, still grinning. "Never ask a lady her age. I apologize."

Mom, apparently placated by the apology, cracked a tight smile. Dad looked immensely proud. The room was warmer. I felt more energetic than I had in hours. All because Mom had given us, and we had taken advantage of, the opportunity to laugh.

Laughing in the face of Alzheimer's. Dad and I did it as we listened to Mom giving Charley-Dog etiquette instructions on the days when she refused to talk at all to us. We laughed every time she commented on my husband's "lovely" hair. The day she opened her mouth and I saw her dentures were in upside down, I smiled when I wanted to cry. Then I fixed them and I laughed. Her poor gums were no longer being bitten by the false teeth. It was victory over a most unlikely adversary! The day Mom smoked a pen, Dad and I smiled to each other. We weren't laughing at her confusion, but merely enjoying the humor of seeing her blow smoke into the room after a long, satisfying draw on a worn-out ballpoint pen.

Humor was an invaluable companion to us as we traveled the Alzheimer's road. Sometimes, Mom was able to join in, her laughter soft and a little tentative, but her eyes growing brighter, her posture relaxing as she looked around and saw only smiles.

I pray you take every opportunity to laugh.

> **You will make it, even through the most difficult times.**

When you need strength, you will have it. When you need words, they will come to you. When there is nothing you can do to help your loved one, she will, against all odds and expectations, help herself. I can't tell you how it happens—who can explain a miracle?—but I can tell you that resolution always comes. So expect it. Look for it.

Your range of vision will be so much wider if you *expect* solutions to the challenges of Alzheimer's. You will find resources and helpers and solace that you won't see if your eyes are closed in despair.

We pray and trust that someday there will be effective treatments for Alzheimer's. Ways to cure it. Even ways to prevent it. Until then, our peace will be in the knowledge that we can help our loved ones through it. **We can.**

* * *

And that's how I leave you: with a prayer for peace. The peace of knowing you can do this. The peace of knowing you're not alone. The peace of knowing the Lord is with you, and where he is, miracles abound.

I have walked the road you walk. I have held a hand very like the one you're holding. I saw miracles. Believe me—you will, too. God bless you.

Printed in the United States
by Baker & Taylor Publisher Services